MW00531891

THE
DOCTOR
WHO
CURES
CANCER

PRAISE FOR EMANUEL REVICI, M.D.

Below are a few thoughts about Dr. Revici expressed over the years by medical doctors, scientists, researchers and patients.

His brilliance as a medical scientist

Dr. Emanuel Revici is the Louis Pasteur of our time—brilliant, innovative, compassionate, and always at the vangaurd of applied research. A man who has lived long enough to see his ideas benefit tens of thousands—a real treasure!

> Gary Null, Ph.D.
> Author, radio talk-show host.
> Considered one of the world's leading authorities on nutrition

There was Hippocrates, there was Galen, and then there was Paracelsus. He is among them.

> Gerhard Schrauzer, Ph.D.
> Professor of Biochemistry
> Internationally recognized cancer researcher.

Emanuel Revici…is widely regarded as an authentic genius of modern medicine. To some he ranks on the order of a Pasteur. [He is] sometimes regarded as the Nikola Tesla of medicine.

> Robert G. Houston
> Award-winning science writer and researcher
> Consultant on alternative cancer therapies for ABC, Metromedia, PBS, and WNBC
> from *Repression and Reform In The Evaluation of Alternative Cancer Therapies*, Project Cure, Inc.

My father, who was the science editor of the American Cancer Society for 25 years, and I met with Dr. Revici for the first time on a summer's day in the mid 1970's. After two hours of discussion, we left and walked down Park Avenue. I said, "I have to confess I didn't understand a word that man said." He said, "I didn't understand one word either, but I am absolutely convinced—that man is a genius."

> Patrick M. McGrady Jr.
> Former Moscow bureau chief for *Newsweek*
> director of CANHELP, a cancer-patient information and referral service

Genius is seeing what everyone else sees and thinking what no one else thinks. Revici is a genius.

> Robert Fishbein, M.D.
> 34-year survivor of terminal brain cancer
> under Dr. Revici's care

Revici is 50 to 100 years ahead of his time in his knowledge of steroids. His work with steroids alone is earth shattering. I'm not fit to tie his shoelaces. In a hundred years people will say, "isn't it a shame the way people treated Revici when he was alive?"

> Morris Mann, M.D.
> Researcher and independent inventor.

I saw his book and a thousand lights went on. It's part of how I think.

> Lynn August, M.D.
> Researcher on the nature of PMS,
> referring to Revici's textbook.

Dr. Revici's work is an excellent example of advances in medicine that are far beyond the scope of orthodox medicine.

> Robert Atkins, M.D.
> Innovative cancer physician
> Author of *Dr. Atkins' New Diet Revolution*

His results with cancer and AIDS

You requested that I look into Dr. Revici's treatment of cancer. This I did, and find it far beyond my wildest expectations.... His results are amazing...

> Louis E. Burns, M.D.

Dr. Revici has cured many people who were otherwise considered incurable. It is my professional opinion that his medicines have worked for many of the patients whose records I have examined.

> Seymour Brenner, M.D., F.A.C.R.
> Former head of the largest cancer radiation oncology
> center in the United States.

I've known him for ten years. I don't know how he does it, but people walk in dead and walk out alive.

John Heller, M.D.
Former head of Sloan-Kettering Memorial
Cancer Center

...I know of no conventional oncologist who can match his results.

Patrick M. McGrady Jr.
from "The Cancer Patient's Quandary",
The Newsday Magazine,

I tracked down over 200 of Dr. Revici's cases. I studied this man's work for 15 years. I refused to write an article about him for ten years until I had absolute proof from my own investigation that [these] patients had cancer...it was his treatment that put them into remisssion, and they were alive and well ten years later.

Gary Null, Ph.D.

Dr. Revici has been working in my laboratory for two years...It is vital that his research be continued without interruption, for the results obtained by Dr. Revici open a multiplicity of new paths to research of all kinds, particularly in the field of cancer.

Roger. Leroux, M.D.
Professor of Pathologic Anatomy
Faculty of Medicine in Paris
Deputy Director of the Institute of Cancer of Villejuif

Dr. Revici's research in lipids and their therapeutic application in HIV and AIDS has proved to be extremely effective—a fact reflected by improvement of "T" lymphocyte counts and clinical conditions as well. His work is definitely promising and opens vast areas of investigation and study in the field.

Carolina Stamu, M.D.

While many European and American Pharmaceutical companies are looking at protease inhibitors and transcriptease, we feel the real good investment lies on the treatment protocols like what you and Dr. Corsello are doing, a model that has positioned James Mobb as the only Southern African Centre getting wheelchaired AIDS patients back to their work places in weeks.

Richard Ngwenya, M.D.
Harare, Zimbabwe
Referring to protocols developed by the Revici
Life Science Center (1997)

When I worked with Revici in the early and mid-eighties, I saw terminal AIDS patients who improved. Some lived almost normal lives.

A.R. Salman, M.D.

There were people who came in who had AIDS who looked like they were at death's door. You came back a month or two later, and the difference in terms of their improvement was just incredible. He didn't rescue them all but, my Lord, he pulled a lot of people out.

Robert Wilden, a Revici patient and
a nine-year victor over cancer of the jaw

His results with drug and alcohol addiction

The results and what we witnessed [were] so unbelievable that the doctor from Municipal Hospital has now gone back on a daily basis in order to continue with this chance to see the miraculous results that have taken place.

Congressman Charles Rangel
U.S. Congressional Select Committee on Crime
Hearing April 1971. Referring to Revici's success
with drug addiction.

All the patients are drug addicts—heavy long-term users… Normally they should be climbing the walls, vomiting incessantly, clutching their bellies in the agony of withdrawal. Despite the assurances they have received, they seem surprised that they aren't suffering. "I feel fine, doctor," they all say, as Dr. Revici questions them. "No problems."

David A. Loehwing, *Barron's* Sept. 11, 1972
Reporting on patients' experiences with Revici's
detoxification methods for drug addiction.

His alleviation of pain without the use of narcotics

I forgot how much pain there is. I was absolutely shocked by the amount of pain that was there at a very good research hospital. They were screaming in the halls. They were lying on the floor tearing up sheets. With Revici, which were really all terminal cases, there was really very little pain.

Lawrence LeShan, Ph.D.
Author of *Cancer as a Turning Point*
Comparing Walter Reed Hospital with Revici's
Trafalgar Hospital.

...in cases of patients afflicted with grave surgical conditions...the results obtained in the most hopeless of cases were always the amelioration of pain, and quite often the progressive disappearance of large tumors. Dr. Revici's research must be continued and fostered, and may change the therapy of tumors completely.

Dr. Chifoliau
Honored Member of Hospitals of Paris
Member of the French Academy of Surgery

...the thing that impressed me more than anything else is the fact that every patient in this institution is free of, or practically free of, pain without the use of narcotics. In my opinion, if he has nothing else, this ability to relieve intractable pain is a great contribution.

C.A. Calhoun, M.D.

His dedication to his patients

I have never seen a more dedicated physician. I have never known before a physician who told every charge nurse in the hospital that if he was needed at any time, by any patient, he should be called and, to my personal knowledge, if he was called at two, three or four in the morning, he was always there within twenty minutes.

Lawrence LeShan, Ph.D.

You could call him at home any day, at any time. We called him three times on Christmas day, including at 6:41 in the morning and 9:14 at night, plus at 6:30 in the evening on Christmas Eve. I kept a tab on all the calls we made. It totaled 437 calls.

Pearce and Allan Hamilton, patients.

Dr. Revici heard about a patient who was too sick to come and see him. He paid the man a house call, walking up five flights of stairs. Revici was ninety-three.

Marcus Cohen
Considered the leading historian
on the life and work of Dr. Revici

His effect on the future of medicine

His lifework is a rich vein of gold waiting to be mined

Dwight L. McKee, M.D.

Whether you are a medical or a non-medical person, when you hear the stories of these cases, when you see the x-rays of bones eaten away by cancer and then returning to normal, how can one but believe? I hope we can get more medical people to see the light and put his treatment into practice.

Louis E. Burns, M.D.

It's not alternative medicine. It's *real* medicine

Carolina Stamu, M.D.

A man who is years ahead of his time—laying the foundation for twenty-first century medicine.

Barry Sears, Ph.D.
Author of *The Zone* and *Mastering The Zone*
Pioneer in developing drug delivery sytems
for cancer and heart patients.

THE DOCTOR WHO CURES CANCER

Sullivan & Foster Publishing, New York
An Entagon Communications Company

Sullivan & Foster Publishing
An Entagon Communications Company
173 West 81st Street
New York, NY 10024

Cover and book design: Alan Barnett, Inc.
Cover photograph: Dan Howell
Index: Marie-Celeste Scully

Library of Congress Cataloging-in-Publication Data

Eidem, William Kelley.
    The doctor who cures cancer / by William Kelley Eidem : foreword by Seymour Brenner. — Rev. ed.
        p. cm.
    Previously published: Bethesda, Md. : Be Well Books, 1996.
    Includes index.
    ISBN 1-890410-01-2 (hardcover)
    1. Revici, Emanuel. 1896–   . 2. Oncologists—United States—Biography. 3. Cancer—Alternative treatment.
    I. Title.
    RC279.6.R48E36   1997
    616.99 '4' 0092—dc21
    [B]   97-13696
                                                            CIP

First edition originally published as *The Man Who Cures Cancer,* Be Well Books, 1996.

Manufactured in the United States of America
Printing (last digit): 10 9 8 7 6 5 4 3 2 1

For my son, Daniel

ERRATA

Alas, in our rush to get this important information to the public, we inadvertently reversed some concepts regarding Dr. Revici's theory of dualism. Four terms are reversed: AM/PM, acid/alkaline, above/below, and anabolic/catabolic on pages 35, 45, 68, 111, 112, and 316 to 322.

Also keep in mind that individual patterns may vary and prior treatments can mask the body's imbalance. As always, for any medical condition, be sure to consult a physician.

DISCLAIMER AND IMPORTANT NOTE TO THE READER

The material in this book is for informational purposes only. The book is not intended to diagnose or treat medical or physical problems and the author and publisher are not engaged in rendering medical services. Before implementing any of the ideas found in this book, or if medical, professional, or other expert assistance is required, the reader is strongly cautioned to consult a physician.

The book is sold without warranties of any kind, expressed or implied, and the publisher and author disclaim any liability, loss or damage caused by the contents of this book. The book is based on information from sources believed to be reliable, and every effort has been made to make the book as accurate as possible. Despite best efforts, however, any errors are the sole responsibility of the author.

Furthermore, the facts, opinions, and choice of title are the responsibility of the author alone, and do not necessarily reflect the opinions or beliefs of the publisher, Emanuel Revici, M.D., his immediate family, or the staff of the Revici Life Science Center.

It is ultimately you, the reader, who must take full responsibility for your well-being and how you use this book.

The author and publisher wish you the very best of health.

Contents

Acknowledgments

This book would not have been possible were it not for the help of a great many people who opened their homes, their hearts and their files to me.

To **Vernon Morin** and his wife, **Judy,** it was your story that led me on this odyssey. Your willingness to spend so much time with me is gratefully remembered.

To **Marcus Cohen,** you were the first person I spoke to at Dr. Revici's office, and a great help during the tough early going.

To **Alice Ladas,** thank you for sharing the many recordings you and your late husband, Professor **Harold Ladas,** made and the letters each of you wrote during Dr. Revici's difficult times. Your generous contribution of time and so much more to Dr. Revici provided a valuable link in this epic saga. Thank-you also for generously providing me with a copy of your manuscript, Veni, Vidi, Revici.

To **Dr. Dwight McKee** for kindly answering my questions, and for speaking out on Revici's behalf when it was so dangerous professionally to do so.

To **Carolyn Gitman,** the 90th birthday bash thrower par excellence, thank you for going through your storage material and sending me the variety of material that you did, especially the meticulously-typed transcripts of radio broadcasts you had recorded.

To **Sam Abady,** that rare lawyer whose personal kindness exceeds even his prodigious court room skills, thank you for making a space for me at your office where I could work for weeks on end. The after-midnight rides in the executive cars also made getting up the next morning that much easier.

To **Richard Jaffe,** another great lawyer, who was kind enough to take my calls in the midst of defending another cancer hero, Stanislaw Burzynski, M.D., thanks for answering my questions and filling me in on some great details.

To **Mirce Panaitescu,** a man whose heart fills whatever room he enters, a devoted family man, and the man who makes the medicines, you have the most important job in the world. I'm sure your devotion makes the medicines that much better.

To **Ruth Spector,** a courageous woman who adds life and laughter wherever she goes, your courageous spirit is a joy to be around.

To **Alex Beau,** who rented me a room for three months that turned into a year-and-a-half. Without your patience, support, and understanding, this book would not have seen the light of day until the next century at the earliest. You made the 18 months easy.

To **Gary Null,** thank you for permitting your staff to go through your old archives and providing me with a video tape of Dr. Revici when he was a young man of 88.

To **Robert Houston,** for generously sharing some of the most impressive information in this whole story.

To **Ethel Pratt,** the woman who over the years has done more than anyone to save Dr. Revici from financial ruin, thank you for all the papers you provided me and for your generosity.

To **Dr. Joe Saunders,** for spending hours addressing envelopes so that I might be able to get in touch with some of Revici's Washington-area patients.

To **Dick Adams,** for kindly digging out and handing me about two feet of files.

To **Dr. Seymour Brenner** and his wife **Phyllis,** for graciously opening your home to me and taking all my calls.

To **Dr. A. R. Salman,** for your warmth and your time, and for answering my dumbest questions.

To Professor **Gerhard Schrauzer,** for letting your love for Dr. Revici and his work overcome your reluctance to speak on his behalf.

To **Dr. Carolina Stamu,** the only physician who has ever offered to fix me a cup of coffee during office hours, thank you for acting as my go-between with Dr. Revici when I was unable to make it to New York.

To **Shirley Cahayom,** the sweetest receptionist a doctor could have, thank you for lunch, for the subway token, and for all your help.

To **Gilbert Saltman,** for generously sharing your knowledge and insightful ideas.

To **Rodika Mihaescu,** for all the photocopying etc., etc.

To **Emil Hara,** for helping Dr. Revici in so many ways that might not be recognized.

To **Dr. Emanuel Revici,** for opening your office, your home, your non-patient files and your sofa bed. You might not have invented kindness, but you have probably improved upon it.

To **Karen Schecter** of Creedmoor State Hospital, thank you for finding the LaBurt and Revici study on schizophrenia from 1949 and mailing me a copy.

To **all the patients** who took my calls and answered my questions, even though I was a stranger to you, thank you. Although there were far too many stories to include all of them, it is because of you and future patients like you that this story is being written.

To the person who asked to remain **anonymous,** but who helped me with a lovely grace and elegance, a special thanks to you.

Foreword

Dr. Emanuel Revici treats cancer in a manner unlike any other doctor in the United States—and probably in the world. He uses his own medicines. Over the years he has developed over 100 different medications in his own laboratory. I don't know how they work, but I have seen their results.

I am a retired board-certified radiation oncologist. My practice specialized in the treatment of cancer with radiation. I have fought at the front lines in the war against cancer all of my professional life. During my long tenure of battling cancer for my patients, I gradually became rather frustrated and unhappy with the little progress that has been made in the treatment of this disease.

After more than forty years of seeing almost no breakthroughs on the medical front, it became painful seeing my patients every day, knowing that most of them had very little chance for a cure. On numerous occasions I saw patients in tears. Just as often I saw wives crying for their husbands, husbands crying for their wives, and parents crying for their sick children.

My combined Brooklyn and Queens offices handled several hundred appointments a week during the last ten years of my practice, making it the largest cancer radiation oncology center in the nation. Highly regarded physicians whose offices were in the shadows of Sloan-Kettering, Columbia University College of Physicians and Surgeons, and NYU Medical Center sent their patients to our offices. I was a member of the Cancer and Acute Leukemia Group "B", which is the largest nationally funded cancer research group in the United States. Our office provided this organization with statistical data regarding our patients.

My practice produced a personal income for me well into the seven figure range annually. For four decades our offices were technologically state-of-the-art. We repeatedly spent millions of dollars in order to procure the latest and best radiation and diagnostic equipment available. Despite that outward success, I am still saddened from having watched so many people of all ages die.

Even with the best possible equipment and a staff of board-certified radiation oncologists, we could only do so much. Sadly, for the population of patients we saw, the odds were against them. Many came to us hoping to be cured. When I examined their records, though, I knew which ones were being treated for a possible cure, and which ones were being treated for palliation (relief of pain).

Since 1950 the medical profession has made only minor advances in the therapeutic arena against cancer. The only significant improvement that I saw was in our diagnostic abilities. As a result, some cancers, such as cancer of the breast, colon, uterus and prostate have cure rates of 90% or better if caught in Stage I.

I must state, however, that these four highly curable cancers become incurable if not caught in their early stages—Stages I or II. Although the overall numbers say you have a fifty-fifty chance of beating cancer, the individual numbers say you either have a 90% chance or very little chance, depending on what stage the cancer is in and its type. Unfortunately, for a few cancers, such as pancreatic cancer, the patient is lucky to live much more than six months regardless of the treatment. Even with the all-out effort to catch cancer earlier than ever before, the overall five-year cure rate has inched up a paltry 0.7% in the last 40 years.

I first became interested in Emanuel Revici, M.D., not from the medical literature, but from hard evidence—that is, x-rays taken at my office of one of my patients. I knew his prior condition because this was a patient we had seen a year earlier. His cancer of the lung had metastasized to his bones.

There was no mistaking the improvement in the patient. When I saw that his new films showed no evidence of cancer either in his bones or lungs, I had to find out what had caused the remission.

The patient told me he had been undergoing treatment by a Dr. Revici in Manhattan. At the time I was unfamiliar with the gentleman. Still I arranged to meet with him at his office. When I first met Dr. Revici, he was already 90 years old. He showed me enough "before" and "after" x-rays and CT scans at our first meeting for me to schedule a second one.

A few days later he introduced me to three patients who had previously been stricken with incurable cancer. Two of them had been afflicted with pancreatic cancer and the other was previously diagnosed with a malignant brain tumor. Dr. Revici showed me their CT scans both before and after his treatment. The "before" pictures showed a suspicious mass for each patient. He also showed me the written biopsy reports from the various hospitals which had confirmed that the abnormal masses were cancerous. The "after" scans showed no evidence of any abnormality. From all outward appearances the three patients looked to be healthy. Dr. Revici also showed me copies of reports from the patients' private physicians who confirmed that the patients were now free of cancer.

I knew from my own training and experience that modern medicine couldn't have saved those three people. Each of the three patients had an almost zero percent chance of recovery. That all three would be free of cancer led me to think that Dr. Revici's medicines were worth further investigation.

Since those early meetings I have reviewed the records, x-rays, CT scans and biopsy reports of dozens of Dr. Revici's patients. Often, when Dr. Revici provided me with information on a patient, I would attempt to confirm it with the patient's previous physician. I soon found out that every time Dr. Revici had provided me with information regarding a patient, it would turn out to be correct.

As a Diplomate of Radiology I have reviewed many cases of incurable cancer that Dr. Revici has cured. I must admit that his results aren't always 100%, but then neither are the results of the approved medical profession 100%.

In my entire career of seeing tens of thousands of patients, I have never seen a single case of spontaneous remission, except for misdiagnosed lung cancer. The cases I reviewed at Dr. Revici's office were not misdiagnosed. In my opinion, it's unlikely that the positive outcomes I reviewed were the result of multiple spontaneous remissions.

I must interject a brief story at this point. When I met Dr. Revici, I was sixty-two years old. My PSA reading, the screening test for prostate cancer, was 6.2. A PSA score of up to 5.0 is normal. Scores from 5.0 to 10.0 need to be watched, as some may indicate the presence of cancer. Above 10.0 there's a greatly elevated chance of cancer.

When I told Dr. Revici about my PSA score, he gave me one of his medications. After taking the medicine for a year, my PSA reading fell to 1.6. There were no apparent ill effects. After a few years of being off the medicine, my latest PSA reading has inched up to 2.5.

After examining the records of a number of his patients, I am now of the opinion that Dr. Revici has something worthy of a thorough clinical trial. I decided to see if I could help Dr. Revici to conduct a large scale test of his method and his medicines.

I made a presentation at a Congressional hearing in March of 1988. At that time I proposed a study to test Dr. Revici's method for treating cancer. Once it is approved, the study will include 100 cases of cancer that the medical profession recognizes as incurable: pancreatic cancer, colon cancer with liver metastases, unresectable lung cancer, and unresectable brain cancer. The patients are to be selected by five board-certified oncologists who will verify that each patient is incurable, and that his or her life expectancy is less than one year.

Sloan-Kettering, NIH, the Mayo Clinic, M. D. Anderson, John Hopkins and many other outstanding research centers accept cancer patients for experimental trials every day. The patients who volunteer often decide to participate because they believe it might give them a chance they might not have otherwise. I believe it's time to conduct an experimental trial of Revici's medicines. These patients would have nothing to lose by their participation. From what I have seen, there is the chance that they would have something to gain.

Dr. Revici has cured many people who were otherwise considered incurable. It is my professional opinion that his medicines have worked for many of the patients whose records I have examined. Let's find out if more patients and their families can be helped.

The fact that he has helped so many people means it's time for Mr. and Mrs. America to push for a clinical trial of his method.

—Seymour Brenner, M. D., F.A.C.R.

Introduction

The Doctor Who Cures Cancer is really about you. It's about having answers to real health questions—even serious ones. Answers you can apply at home literally as easily as breathing. It's also about several unifying discoveries made by Emanuel Revici, M.D. that are so deceptively simple you'll actually understand how your body came to be put together in the way that it is. You'll also learn several simple keys about becoming healthier, even if you are quite sick. In some respects, as strange as it may sound, you will have a better understanding of the fundamental mechanisms of sickness and health than many of today's health care professionals.

But *The Doctor Who Cures Cancer* is also about our medical community and its ability to assimilate new scientific information that in many cases can be lifesaving. As you read through this book you will be amazed at the medicines and treatments that Dr. Revici has not only discovered, but also applied to thousands of patients with remarkable success. And you will be fascinated with the paradigm shifts of Revici's thinking—all based on the rock-solid principles of physics, chemistry, and biochemistry. Yet the acknowledgment he received from the medical community has been nothing short of shameful.

But first, you should know that small but significant portions of Dr. Revici's long-suppressed discoveries are beginning to seep into the public's awareness. Entire books have been written, in fact, which have unknowingly profited from similar or identical ideas developed and researched by Dr. Revici generations ago. For example, the scientific cornerstone of Dr. Barry Sears' New York Times bestseller, *The Zone*, is based on a principle which, for Dr. Revici, was just one single aspect of his many discoveries.*

Another New York Times bestseller, *The Arthritis Cure*, advises readers to use glucosamine as a key part of its program to reverse arthritis. Its authors cite several different studies on glucosamine research, the earliest of which was published in 1980. Dr. Revici first used glucosamine as a replacement for steroids in the treatment of arthritis in his patients beginning in 1951. Dr. Revici wrote about his findings ten years later in his textbook published in 1961. In fact, you will discover that Dr. Revici had achieved results long ago in the treatment of arthritis that sometimes exceed those discussed in *The Arthritis Cure*, especially with rheumatoid arthritis. *(The Arthritis Cure* offers no breakthrough in the treatment of rheumatoid arthritis, whereas Dr. Revici's approach has produced quite positive results in the treatment of that condition for several decades.)

As useful as those books are, they merely peek into a much deeper body of work. With this book you'll have insights into and, in many cases, answers for the major diseases such as cancer, AIDS, heart disease, arthritis, depression, alcoholism and so on—all based on science, not speculation. In addition, you'll learn about real medicine that not only controls cancer and other diseases, but actually gets rid of them. And you won't have to rely on a strict diet to obtain help.

Wouldn't you like to have access to medications without side effects that could actually make bones attacked by cancer grow back while simultaneously making your pain vanish?

Wouldn't you like it if you (or a loved one) had cancer, AIDS, arthritis, depression or asthma, and you could be able to monitor your

---

* Dr. Barry Sears, in his monumental best-selling book, *The Zone*, has uncannily and apparently unknowingly made use of a small portion of Dr. Revici's discoveries. Dr. Sears refers to the Nobel-Prize-winning work of Bengst Samuelsson as the scientifically-grounded basis for part of his own findings. In fact, Sears emphasizes that his reliance on that discovery is the scientific cornerstone of his dietary theory. According to A. R. Salman, M.D., Samuelsson's findings, made in the mid 1970's, are one and the same as Dr. Revici's overlooked discovery made in the mid 1940's. Dr. Salman has said repeatedly that Revici's earlier work in this area is "clearer and more detailed" than Samuelsson's.

progress at home?

If you were feeling a little under the weather with a headache or other malady, wouldn't it be great if you could check out your acid/alkaline balance in just seconds *simply by exhaling?*

Wouldn't you like to have access to real anti-viral medications for such things as colds, flus, pneumonia—even AIDS and Ebola?

Wouldn't you like to see medications that could remove drug and alcohol addiction quickly and effectively without side effects or withdrawal?

You can. They have existed for nearly 30 years—thanks to Dr. Revici.

But surely, if any of that was possible, we would have heard of them before or, at the very least, organized medicine would be taking advantage of Dr. Revici's discoveries. In this book you will learn the sad details of how the seemingly impossible task of keeping these medicines from most of the general public for half a century has been achieved.

You'll also discover, however, that organized medicine has been incorporating principles of Revici's work for years—only they don't know it! Today there is a lifesaving medication to speed up the development of premature babies' lungs that is used by physicians across the land. Its genesis comes directly from one of the fundamental tenets of Dr. Revici's original textbook, *Research In Physiopathology*, first published in 1961 and recently brought back into print.

When Drs. John Clements and Julius Comroe isolated the lipid responsible for that mechanism, they had no idea that Dr. Revici had already been applying that principle for many years. Nor did they know that the seed for their discovery came from Revici himself. Common medicine still hasn't caught up with the far-reaching ramifications of that work, which includes effective treatments for invasive cancer. It is also likely that if Revici's name had been attached to the Clements/Comroe discovery, it never would have seen the light of day Why? Because doing so would have required acknowledgment and acceptance of the Revici Method itself.

On Christmas day of 1996, the Journal of the American Medical Association (JAMA) published the results of a major study which demonstrated the remarkable effects of selenium in halving lung and colon cancer incidence and deaths. Dr. Revici began using selenium effectively in the treatment of cancer in 1954. While the editors of JAMA still struggle with the toxicity problems associated with selenium, Revici easily solved that challenge more than four decades earlier. Despite the prejudice towards the man, his findings are beginning to take hold in the form of basic medical knowledge and practice among physicians. Emanuel Revici's name might be controversial in the high halls of common medicine, but his discoveries are diamonds. As a reader, you will be able to select the gems of your choosing.

A few scientists already have. The former University of San Diego Professor Gerhard Schrauzer, an internationally recognized mainstream cancer researcher, has recently compared Dr. Revici to Hippocrates and Paracelsus. One physician-turned-inventor, who is also a longtime expert in steroids, has said that Dr. Revici is 50 to 100 years ahead of his time just in his knowledge of those substances. In 1961, a group of world-renowned scientists that includes 14 Nobel prize winners was similarly impressed, so they awarded Dr. Revici their prestigious annual medal. As far back as 1955, a physician was asked by a businessman who was considering supporting Revici's research in cancer to look into it. After researching it, Dr. Louis E. Burns wrote the following.

> You requested that I look into Dr. Revici's treatment of cancer. This I did, and find it beyond my wildest expectations.... His results are amazing.

What I have attempted to do is to provide some of the most important discoveries that Revici has made in a form that can be understood and used by you, the reader. Since I am very much a lay person, you will find that I don't use a lot of technical verbiage or scientific jargon. Still, I was pleased to hear from one physician who is familiar with Dr. Revici's work and who had read the manuscript. She said that it helped her to understand his approach even more than she already did.

People often ask me how I, a freelance writer, came upon this story. Quite simply, I was interviewing Congressman Peter DeFazio of Oregon who told me about a bill he had introduced in the House of

Representatives called "The Access to Medical Treatment Act." He also told me about a hearing on it that had taken place in the Senate two weeks earlier. One of the witnesses at the Senate subcommittee hearing was Vernon Morin, who testified on behalf of his five-year-old daughter, Issy. His testimony was stunning. (You'll meet Issy within these pages.) After a two-hour, long-distance conversation regarding Dr. Revici's work, I met Vernon on his small farm in southern New Jersey. Since that time, as the facts have unfolded, the story has exceeded any expectations I might have had. (If you haven't read Dr. Seymour Brenner's foreword yet, you are in for an eye-opening essay.)

My first meeting with Dr. Revici took place on September 13, 1994, exactly one week after his 98th birthday. The memory of seeing him as I walked down a hallway has stayed with me ever since. There sat a tiny man with a small, peaceful smile from behind a huge desk. On the walls were two framed Periodic Tables of the Chemical Elements. One was to his left. Towards the bottom of it, was a large color drawing of its originator, the Russian chemist, Dmitry Mendeleyev.

The other chart was on the wall behind him to his right. It had been sent to him by some medical students from Germany. The chart was entitled, "The Revici Periodic Table" (see appendix B). This book is the first to explain in plain English the dramatic impact of Revici's new look at an old chart.

A few of the many people I have interviewed suggested that I be careful not to make Revici out to be a saint. Yet, at the same time, they stressed that he is exceedingly generous and kind. From my own research it appears that his many virtues exceed his few weaknesses—probably more so than is true for most of us. I believe you will see that as you read on.

The central focus of this book concerns much more significant matters—at least from a medical standpoint. It is about a man who has devoted nearly every waking hour of his long life to making illness less of a burden for people. Because that has been his focus, I have attempted to do the same by concentrating mostly on his work and his many discoveries. In addition I have translated some of those principles so you can apply them personally if you wish.

Since that first visit I have spoken with him on numerous occasions. Based on audio tapes of some talks from the mid-1980's, it is clear that his advanced age causes him to speak in simpler terms than when he was younger. As a result some of these quotes will be in simple language—or even in somewhat broken English—while others are not. Although his syntax might not always be textbook, you'll see that his thoughts are to the point. When I was interviewing him, I found the simplicity of his expression often added to its impact. Therefore, I have chosen to share with you his own words, unfiltered by a grammar text. Revici didn't learn to speak English (his sixth language) until he was almost fifty years old. Yet his written command of the English language, based on some of his documents, indicates that it was frequently rather good.

Dr. Revici is a man whose energy has seldom waned. Much of his creative work is done between the hours of midnight and eight o'clock in the morning. On nights when I have been a guest at his five-room, elegantly-modest Park Avenue apartment in Manhattan, I have seen him in the middle of the night working and pondering. On one occasion, around two or three in the morning, he said, "You get some sleep, I am working."

That habit of reading, pondering and writing in the middle of the night from midnight until morning is something he has done all his adult life and apparently even as a child. Perhaps most remarkable of all was his ability to hold a document six inches from his face, reading it without glasses. Although he has glasses, he didn't seem to need them—but then, he was only ninety-eight years old at the time. He now needs a cane and a helping hand to walk from place to place, reportedly due to the ravages of a serious food poisoning that settled into his hip from bad pork he had eaten more than a half-century ago.

Yet the years that have exacted a physical toll have had less effect on his mind. Even now, at the top of his bed, are hundreds if not thousands of small squares of papers bound in rubber bands or in paper clips with notations that he has made. The middle drawer of his office desk is similarly filled with bound notes on various medical topics. When he was shown an old article referring to work he did with schizophrenics nearly fifty years ago, he pointed repeatedly at a particular line in the paper with his finger and said, "This makes me think of something entirely new, I must work on it." That tireless devotion to a single cause for more than 80 years, coupled with a brilliant mind and a caring heart, has produced a most remarkable treasure of over 100 medicines for the treatment of cancer, AIDS, smoking, drug addiction, alcoholism, arthritis, depression, schizophrenia, heart disease, high blood pressure, migraines, cuts and burns, asthma, childhood retardation, herpes, colitis and many other conditions.

Within these pages you will meet some of the people he has helped. Their stories are living proof that Dr. Revici's medicines aren't alternative medicine—but real medicine.

There are many books that tell how and why a certain discovery changed society. This book tells you history in advance. After you have read *The Doctor Who Cures Cancer*, you will be able to watch history unfold from a vantage point seldom available. But more importantly, you will have information that can help you take advantage of Dr. Revici's discoveries should you or your family ever need it.

P.S. About the title and the word "cure": Dr. Revici and I have different perspectives about what constitutes the cure of cancer in a patient. Dr. Revici's position is quite clear. All of his life he has repeatedly said that with cancer patients one can never be sure if every last cancer cell has been eradicated. Consequently, he has steadfastly held that one can never say a cancer is cured. For example, not once in his own 773-page book did Dr. Revici ever claim a patient to be cured of cancer, although the temptation might have been great considering the results he had achieved. Furthermore, Revici has avoided ever saying any of his patients were cured of cancer regardless of how long they have lived without a recurrence of the symptoms.

Dr. Revici is much more conservative than the American Cancer Society (ACS) in respect to what constitutes a cure. The ACS generally considers a patient cured if he or she survives five years beyond the initial diagnosis regardless of the patient's condition at the end of those five years. The American Cancer Society refers to cancer as one of the most curable of the major diseases. The organization will also admit it doesn't know what the mechanism of cancer is. How they can reconcile those contradictory stances is left to them to explain. Some cancer researchers have held that cancer cells are always present in the human body but are held in check by some as yet not fully understood mechanism. If cancer cells are always present, then we must differentiate between a dormant cancer cell and an active cancer cell.

A metaphor from nature might help to differentiate between cancer and a malignancy. A resting lion with a full stomach is of little danger to a group of zebras, but a lion in pursuit is a different story entirely. With that concept in mind, the question of what is a fair definition for curing cancer might fall somewhere between Dr. Revici's viewpoint and the position of the American Cancer Society.

My American Heritage Dictionary defines the word "cure" as, "1. Restoration of health; recovery from disease. 2. A method or course of treatment used to restore health. 3. An agent, such as a drug, that restores health." In the verb form, the dictionary states, "To restore to health. To get rid of, to remedy." There are many cases in this book that would seem to fit those dictionary definitions. Based upon those dictionary meanings, although Dr. Revici has always refrained from describing himself as a physician who cures cancer, maybe we should. Another title considered for the book was "Real Medicine". That title might better describe the contents of the book since this story is only partially a biography and cancer is only one of the conditions Revici has had success in treating. But the real problem with treating cancer isn't the lack of effective medicines; it's the mistaken belief that truly effective treatments for cancer have not been developed yet. Perhaps the selected title will help correct that mistaken belief. "Real Medicine" doesn't do that, unfortunately.

The final chapter, however, is called "Real Medicine". I hope you enjoy it.

THE DOCTOR WHO CURES CANCER

Issy and the Spider Leg

"You requested that I look into Dr. Revici's treatment of cancer. This I did, and find it far beyond my wildest expectations.... His results are amazing..."

LOUIS E. BURNS, M.D., 1955

"We can cure this disease if we can get a national effort behind it"

SAM DONALDSON, ABC NEWS, 1996, IN AN INTERVIEW
WITH LARRY KING ABOUT CANCER.

Two weeks before little Issy was taken to see Emanuel Revici, M.D., in Manhattan, her doctors at Children's Hospital of Philadelphia (CHOP) had estimated she had two or possibly three weeks left to live.

Five hundred thousand dollars of prior medical treatments had not cured her because a grapefruit-sized tumor pressed against the four-year-old's large intestine and liver. Meanwhile, the malignant growth had sprouted a six-foot predatory spider leg that wrapped itself around her spine. In addition, one of her chemotherapy sessions at CHOP had injured her kidneys and bladder, according to her father, Vernon Morin.

The Morins were cautioned by Issy's doctors that their daughter would probably die a painful death, although they would prescribe some narcotics to try to reduce her pain. The only "good" news they had to offer was that the end would come quickly.

Her parents would not give up, however. Two days after starting Dr. Revici's treatment, Issy's pain disappeared, so she no longer needed any pain killers. The first office visit cost less than $200. The medicine was free.

Issy spent that summer playing and swimming in the river behind her parent's home. As her treatment continued, she gained weight, began to grow, returned to preschool, and started ballet classes. Her sweet and playful disposition returned as well.

After nine months of Revici's care, Issy's grapefruit-sized tumor was smaller than a golf ball. The dangerous spider leg was dead. Where tests had previously shown 98% cancer cells in her peripheral blood, now there were none.

Meanwhile—when no one else could help Issy Morin—the state of New York yanked Dr. Revici's medical license.

Nor was Issy's battle over. The long-term effects of her kidney damage caused her to go into shock. But the people who said Issy would only last a few weeks had not referred her to a kidney specialist. Issy could overcome the cancer, but like Revici, she was no match for the medical establishment. Five months after her first coma, Issy surrendered for the last time.

Was it just luck that caused Issy's tumor to shrink so much? Why did the invasive spider leg shrivel up and go away? Well, consider that the 100-year-old Dr. Revici has had six decades of success with cancer patients who have benefited from his discoveries. Those patients were just as lucky and just as spontaneously healed as little Issy, for Dr. Revici is the doctor who cures cancer.

More than thirty years ago, Dr. John Heller, who was then the medical director of Sloan-Kettering Memorial Cancer Center, privately said of Dr. Revici, "I've known him for ten years. I don't know how he does it, but people walk in dead and walk out alive." This is the story of that man and his many lucky patients, and of a medical establishment that has fought him every step of the way.

Who is Dr. Revici, what has he discovered, and why do his patients consider him to be a miracle worker? Furthermore, how did the forces of conventional medicine stop him from helping the vulnerable Issies of the world?

Perhaps more importantly, what do Revici's discoveries mean for the future of cancer treatment and other conditions, such as AIDS and drug addiction, and how can we personally benefit from his work? The answers to those questions—and more—start with an exploding ambulance.

PART

I

HIS LIFE

1

Living with the Nazis Overhead

"Get out! Drop everything and run!"

PARIS CHIEF OF POLICE
IN A TELEPHONE CALL TO DR. REVICI

*"There was Hippocrates, there was Galen,
and then there was Paracelsus. He is among them."*

PROFESSOR GERHARD SCHRAUZER,
SPEAKING OF DR. REVICI

Emanuel Revici was born over a century ago, a century apart from this one, in the plains of a mountainous country that was also a kingdom, in a land without telephone or radio, but with a culture that rivals our own. On September 6, 1896, from that land of simplicity and royalty, of farmers and kings, in Bucharest, Romania, was born perhaps the greatest medical scientist this world has ever known.

Some memories fade with the passage of a century of life. Still, there are a few that have stayed with Dr. Revici and that seem to have influenced his entire life. At the age of ninety-eight Dr. Revici told me about a few of them. His father, Tullius Revici, M.D., was a physician

3

whose practice ranged from members of the nobility to the local peasantry. Emanuel showed an early spark of interest in his father's profession. "My father had a microscope. We started playing," Dr. Revici would tell me. Because of Emanuel's interest, Tullius and his son had many conversations about the practice of medicine.

As a boy Emanuel seemed to need little sleep and would often stay up half the night. He sometimes watched curiously as his father would go out late at night to see patients. Once, when Emanuel was young, he waited for his father's return and asked him how much he was paid for the long, late-night house call. Tullius told his son he had not charged the patient because the family had little money. It was a lesson Emanuel would remember and would put into practice during his entire professional career.

When Emanuel was ten, he told his father he wanted to be a physician. Tullius asked him why he would want to follow in his father's footsteps. Emanuel told him, "I want to help people."

His father pushed him on his answer, "Is it because you also think you can make a good living?"

"No, I want to help people, only that," Emanuel answered.

Tullius was finally satisfied, "I'm glad you answered this way. If you had told me you also wanted to make a lot of money, I would have been disappointed."

At the age of twelve, Emanuel took on the task of writing four medical books about the human body. He said he stopped at the fifth book, which would have been about the brain, because he found it too difficult. His father told him he was too young to be writing about such things, although one might guess he was secretly pleased.

Emanuel's apparent intelligence and his interest in medicine could not be denied for long, however. By the age of sixteen he began to attend the Bucharest School of Medicine—a full four years ahead of the average first-year student.

Revici was pulled out of his fourth year of medical school to serve as a field doctor in what would become World War I. He saw many soldiers die. "The trenches were dug in a straight line," he said, "so one shell killed many."

Seventy-five years later Revici recounted a story of an event that would change his life. On a day like so many others, his squad traveled down a road with their horse-drawn ambulances. In addition to himself, his ambulance carried a medic and a wounded soldier. He called for the caravan to stop. Lieutenant Revici climbed out and went off into the woods to relieve himself. Within seconds the group was attacked, and at least one shell hit his ambulance. Both men inside were killed, as was the man riding on top of the ambulance. The two horses that were hitched to the ambulance were also killed in the shelling.

After Revici returned to Bucharest and the story was told, he was taken off this front-line detail and reassigned to the hospital—possibly because he was so young, or perhaps because his intelligence was recognized as something that should not be lost.

He found himself in trouble almost right away. Revici, who specialized in bacteriology while in medical school, quickly realized that too-high a number of patients were dying from apparent infection. He performed some pathological autopsies on a few of the dead and found that the cause of death was cholera, a condition that was believed to have been previously eradicated.

His discovery did not sit well with certain higher-ups. Fortunately, even at his early age, Revici had gained the respect of some of the more senior people at the hospital, including Professor D. Danielopolu, chairman of medicine and a member of the French Academy, who said, "I know Dr. Revici. His specialty is bacteriology. If he says it's cholera, then that's what it is." Through further investigation, Revici was able to track down the probable source of the outbreak to a patient from a remote area who had come in contact with some refugees from Russia.

When the war ended, Revici returned to medical school, from where he would graduate at the top of his class in 1920. Because of his number-one class ranking, he was automatically offered a teaching position at the university. He accepted the offer and within a few years he would become an assistant professor there.

Revici also opened his own medical practice. His father's habit of treating whoever needed his services would become a hallmark of Dr.

Revici's practice. In seventy-four years as a practicing physician, he would never turn away any patient because he or she was too sick or too poor.

Like his father before him, his patients came from all walks of life. At first his patients would include the farmers and villagers of Romania. His willingness to treat the poor would continue throughout his life. Yet, like his father, the well-to-do also came to see him. Years later he would treat more than three thousand drug addicts, most of whom were from Harlem. In the meantime, he also treated some of the world's luminaries including Oscar winners Anthony Quinn and Gloria Swanson; the Broadway star Gertrude Lawrence; the Archbishop of Ephesus, Lorenzo Michelle DeValich; the Dalai Lama; the wife of the Russian ambassador to Mexico; and the sister of a close advisor to the president of France.

Yet as much as he loved his patients, he also had a deeply curious mind. Throughout most of his life he slept only two to four hours a night. During his waking hours he devoted himself to trying to find answers to the scientific questions that perplexed him. As Dr. A. R. Salman, a former Revici associate, who is now the chief physician of Emerald Coast Hospital in Florida, would recently say, "He didn't go out to movies or dance. He devoted seven days a week, all of his life to his patients, his family and his research."

The incident that precipitated his lifelong work in cancer came from a most unlikely series of events. During his time as a professor, Revici saw on the operating table a young, pregnant woman, surgically opened up, whose abdomen was full of cancer. The operating surgeon closed her up, thinking she didn't have long to live. Dr. Revici never expected to see her alive again.

Two years later, in 1928, the apparently healthy woman returned to see Revici with her small child. The flabbergasted assistant professor wondered how it was possible for the woman to still be alive. The mystery would not leave his mind. He thought and thought about it—a task he is very good at.

Several patients have commented on Revici's ability to literally submerge himself in their charts. He becomes quiet and looks slightly downward, sometimes closing his eyelids, as if he were constructing something in mid-air right in front of his eyes. Whether he used the same approach to ponder the mystery of the pregnant woman is not known. Still, the question that occurred to no one else became his primary interest.

He knew that neither exploratory surgery nor pregnancy by themselves would have a curative effect on the course of a malignant tumor, so he theorized about the possibility that her dramatic recovery was due to the simultaneous occurrence of both events.

He began to study the placenta and noticed that it was rich in fat-soluble products called lipids. He then experimented with animals, testing different placental lipids to see if they would have any effect on the course of cancer. Those lipids produced some tumor reductions for short periods of time, but the tumor growth would often return. In other cases, the lipids produced an increase in tumor activity.

He went to the literature to learn what he could about lipids, but found that there was very little written about them. That did not stop him, however. He devoted what spare time he could to the question— usually in the dead of night. Meanwhile, he continued handling his professorial duties and caring for his patients in his successful medical practice.

Revici's active mind would lead him in other directions as well. He developed a method for purifying motor oil that was far superior to anything available at the time. The process was especially good for the higher purification requirements necessary to produce aviation quality oil. As Dr. Salman has said with awe, "The man *knows* some chemistry."

He knew chemistry so well that he was offered the equivalent of five million dollars by an oil company for the patent. Revici decided to hold on to the patent. With the help of relatives, a small oil refinery was started, "It cost us about six *lei* per liter, and we received fifty-six *lei* for it." The new product was called "Revoil". Revici lost much of his income from his invention during the second World War. With the Communist takeover of Romania after the war, he no longer received any income from it. The Revoil process continues to be used today— to refine both aviation and automobile motor oils.

The income derived from Revoil gave Revici the freedom to go to Paris to further his cancer research. He left for Paris in 1936. He was followed by his wife, Dida, the following year. Their daughter, Nita, who had learned French while attending a Romanian boarding school, joined them in Paris in 1938 at the age of nine. According to Nita, now a medical editor with a Ph.D. in physiology, "We were living in one spacious room. My father came home for dinner. He took me to school. It was quite wonderful. I had both my parents."

While still in Bucharest, Dr. Revici was an avid art collector and would put up different paintings in the patient lounge at the beginning of each new season. When Dida joined her husband in France, the house was boarded up, with all the valuables crated and stored in the house. A year or two later they received a report from one of their relatives that the house had been entered and the crates opened. All of their valuables, including the paintings, were stolen.

Meanwhile in Paris, possibly due to introductions made by Professor Danielopolu, Dr. Revici gained access to several laboratories in which to conduct his research. His work became quite fruitful.

The Pasteur Institute was the most important and prestigious medical center in the world at that time and today remains one of the world's leading medical research institutes. The competition to get scientific papers published at the Institute was extremely high. In 1937 Revici submitted five papers on lipids and cancer to the Pasteur Institute with the hope that the Institute would consider publishing one of them. All five were accepted—two in 1937 and three in 1938. His reputation soared as a result, and he was called upon by numerous doctors to treat some of their most difficult cases.

In the course of being invited to treat other physicians' patients, Revici was offered the French Legion of Honor. The offer came as a result of his reversing the cancer of the wife of an advisor to the president of France. Revici declined to accept the honor, because he felt that such honors were political in nature.

A second offer of a French Legion of Honor would come as well. Revici had turned over to the French government the patents to a number of his inventions with the idea that they were to be used in the fight against the invading Nazis. Once again, Revici declined the honor.

While Nita was away at a camp during the Summer of 1939, Revici had a serious lab accident, jabbing himself with a needle containing an aggressive virus. The virus settled in the part of Dr. Revici's brain that controlled his breathing. He was placed into an iron lung, and his chances for a complete recovery were dim. He rallied, however, and was released.

The illness has never entirely left Dr. Revici. For the past twenty years he has developed pneumonia at least once a year, probably as a result of the lab accident. Fortunately, he has always had his own anti-viral medicines with which to treat himself. So far, the 100-year-old patient has pulled through each time.

Dr. Salman reports of a time when Dr. Revici was in his mid-eighties and sick with pneumonia. Revici insisted that Dr. Salman give him an injection of one of the lipid medications. Within 15 minutes he began to improve. After 24 hours Revici had completely recovered. More about Revici's anti-viral medications will be discussed in later chapters.

Meanwhile, with Nita still away at summer camp, Dr. Revici's close friends, Gaston and Nenette Merry, invited Dida and the ailing Emanuel to stay at their summer house outside of Paris at Fontainebleau. Because the air was fresh and clean, they thought it might help his recovery. Not wanting to worry their daughter about her father's condition, her parents hadn't told her of their temporary relocation.

Meanwhile, the administrators of Nita's boarding camp heard rumblings of an imminent German invasion and promptly decided to send all their students home early. Nita wired her father, not knowing of the illness that had befallen him, to request that he pick her up at the Paris train station. Nita's parents never saw the telegram, however.

When she got to the train station, she waited and waited for her father. Finally, Nita was taken to the home of the woman who ran the camp and who had accompanied her to Paris. From there Nita called her father on the telephone.

Almost miraculous good fortune prevented a potential tragedy.

Revici answered the phone just as he was just about to leave the apartment. He had just come back to get some blankets because of the cool night air in the country. It had been his first trip back to the Paris apartment in several weeks. If he hadn't been there at that exact moment, eleven-year-old Nita would have been at a loss, with no idea of where to find her mother and father.

After a period of time known as "the phony war" the Germans outsmarted the French military and outflanked the Maginot Line in their invasion of France, putting Paris at imminent risk. Still, Nita's parents decided to remain for the time being in Paris. In the autumn of 1939 Nita was sent to La Rochelle in southwestern France with her twenty-three-year-old cousin, Fanita, to place them out of danger.

Unfortunately, La Rochelle happened to be the home of a French arsenal and naval center, and, as such, the city became a frequent target for the German air force. According to Nita, "The bombs went boom, boom, boom every night. We spent the nights underground listening to the terror above."

Because of the imminent Nazi invasion of Paris by the Germans, Nita's parents notified Fanita that they would drive to La Rochelle to reunite with her and Nita. From there they would all make their way to Nice. Although Paris and La Rochelle were but a day or two's journey apart, ten days passed with no sight of Nita's parents. Meanwhile, Fanita and Nita saw newsreels that showed German aircraft strafing and killing people on the roads as they tried to flee Paris. Because they received no word from her aunt and uncle, the newsreels led Fanita to believe that they might have been two of the many casualties of the German onslaught. She decided that she and her younger cousin should leave for Nice by train on their own.

But as the two cousins were packing to leave, they heard some loud horns honking. They looked and saw the Revicis' dusty blue Fiat and the Merrys' big car, wearing a mattress as a makeshift helmet. The car was driven by the solitary Nenette because her husband, Gaston, had been called to serve in the French army. A third car in the caravan was occupied by one of Dr. Revici's cancer patients and her husband. The woman was determined not to leave Revici's care. The two-day trip had taken several days longer than expected because the group had chosen to avoid the main roads.

Since the advancing German forces were only a day behind them, the small caravan drove that night without using their headlights towards the town of Saint Fort sur le Ne. Once they arrived they were told of a woman who owned a huge home outside the town. The Revicis found the home to be not much smaller than a minor castle.

The woman who lived there, glad to have a physician stay in her home, invited the Revicis, Fanita and Nenette to stay in one wing. "It was primitive but wonderful. It had a big fireplace and a cauldron that swung from the fireplace," reports Nita. "People soon found out my father was a doctor, so he treated them, and they gave him rabbits and chickens in return. There was nothing to do, so my father, with the assistance of Mrs. Merry, would inoculate the animals and conduct experiments in a shed behind the house."

The two families were soon joined by the Nazis. The occupying German troops set up camp in the town, and the commanding officers decided to use the giant residence as their headquarters. According to Nita, "The lady of the house welcomed them and invited them to stay on the floor above us. We had three German soldiers living right above us tramping about with their heavy boots. They didn't know we were Jews, and we didn't advertise that fact." About two weeks later Gaston returned after being demobilized from the French army.

Because fuel was difficult to obtain for their cars, the Revicis and the Merrys purchased some bicycles to use for running errands around town. After a short while they were able to obtain enough fuel, so with the fighting having subsided, they decided to head back to occupied Paris. The Revici family remained in Paris for a little more than a year, where Dr. Revici continued his research as best he could.

During this time both he and Gaston became very active in the French Resistance. Revici wanted to use his knowledge of chemistry to poison the salt served to the German troops in Paris. Because there was a concern that it might end up poisoning the French people, however, the idea was ultimately abandoned.

Before leaving Paris for the final time, Dr. Revici took some photographs of German positions which he planned to send out of the country. At some point either the Germans or the French sympathizers got wind of it, and everyone was searched, including Dr. Revici. He had the film in his pants pocket. Before he was searched, he stuck his hands into them. When he was told to put his hands into the air, he cupped the small roll beneath his curled fourth and fifth fingers. The soldiers performing the search were so intent on examining his clothes and pockets, they never looked up at his outstretched hands. According to Nita, had they discovered the film, her father probably would have been shot immediately. Soon after, Dr. Revici was able to turn the film over to some British citizens to pass on to their government.

Because of his activity with the French underground, Dr. Revici had befriended others who were doing likewise. One evening in March of 1941, a phone call to Dr. Revici came from the chief of police of Paris. "Get out! Drop everything and run! They are going to arrest you tomorrow," he warned. Of course, the Revicis prepared to leave immediately. The Merrys decided to leave with them. After a train ride with only overnight cases, the two families still needed to cross a dangerous no-man's-land that divided the German-occupied land from free France. The zone, a partially wooded, rural area, was frequently patrolled by German soldiers ready to shoot anyone who tried to cross it.

On Easter morning a mercenary took them along the edge of the forest with six other men and a woman with a tiny infant. They heard a German patrol off in the distance. As Nita tells it, "We rushed into the woods and hid among the leaves. The baby started to cry." According to Nita, one of the men told the mother to quiet the child, "or we will kill it." Fortunately, the baby took to its mother's breast and quieted down.

They knew they would have to make a run for it before the next armed patrol came. But the frightened forty-six-year-old Dida, unaccustomed to running, collapsed with an angina attack. Her husband and Gaston each held her under her armpits as they dragged her through the open field for nearly two miles before they reached free France.

From there the group hired a farmer who took them to another train station in his horse-drawn cart. They changed trains in Lyon on their way to their final destination of Nice. Once there, Dida stayed in bed for several months with worsening angina pains. Meanwhile, Dr. Revici and Gaston reinvolved themselves with the resistance movement.

Both families wanted to emigrate to the United States. Because Gaston was an executive with DuPont, the Merrys possessed U.S. visas. The Revici family did not, however. For the next six months Revici was unsuccessful in obtaining a visa for the U.S. despite the fact that Fanita herself held a low level position with the U.S. embassy: "One of my jobs was to advise people standing in the long lines each day that they had no chance of obtaining permission to enter the United States, unless they already had visas."

Once again good fortune smiled on the Revicis. By chance, on the streets of Nice, Fanita bumped into a former classmate of hers from years earlier. It so happened that Fanita's friend had become the wife of the Mexican Consul. Fanita took advantage of the fortuitous meeting. She explained to her former classmate about her uncle's inability to gain a U.S. visa and asked her if she wouldn't arrange for him to meet with her husband. Fanita told her friend about the important research her uncle was conducting and told her, "A scientist like him shouldn't die here." A meeting was quickly arranged.

When I asked about the topic of conversation that Dr. Revici and the consul must have had, Fanita replied, "There was only one topic Mantzi* was interested in—his work. It was an interview to see if he was worth saving."

Both Nita and Fanita said Dr. Revici and the Consul developed instant rapport with each other. "He was such a charmer; the Consul fell in love with him," Nita said. Thus, with the support of the Mexican Consul during a few months of bureaucracy and diplomatic protocol, the Revicis received their visas, not to the U.S., but to Mexico.

---

* 'Mantzi' is a Romanian nickname for Emanuel and was favored by his relatives. An amateur artist, Dr. Revici also signs his works by that name.

With visas finally in hand, Dr. Revici set out to purchase passage on an ocean liner. The tickets cost a wartime price of $1,000 in gold per person—an outrageous price at that time, except that the war made nothing outrageous by comparison. Despite the dear price, they were able to come up with the fee, possibly from Revoil money or with the help of the Merrys.

To connect with the ship leaving Lisbon, Portugal, the Revicis traveled through Marseilles, France, as well as Barcelona and Madrid, Spain. Prior to reaching Barcelona, their daily diet usually consisted of a hot tomato, a rutabaga and some bread made from flour and wood shavings. A monthly egg completed their diet while in Nice. "I remember once my mother giving me one little cube of sugar when I came home from school," Nita recalled.

Food was not quite so scarce in Barcelona, so they went to a restaurant to eat well for the first time in quite a while. Not long after they had begun to eat, they couldn't help but notice some children outside the restaurant. According to Nita, "Small, hungry children stood with their faces against the glass to watch us eat." Their sympathies immediately outweighed their own hunger. Nita and her father took what remained of their food and, "gave it to the children."

The Cunnard Lines ship for which they had purchased their expensive tickets had left before the Revicis were able to arrive. Dr. Revici and his family were, of course, furious and upset with the terrible turn of events. Unknown to them at the time, missing the ship turned out to be another example of their good luck. They learned later that the ship was sunk by a Nazi U-boat.

Fortunately, the tickets were honored by another ship departing a few days later. The Portuguese-flagged Quanza then left for Casablanca, Morocco on the northern coast of Africa to pick up some Spanish military leaders and government cabinet members of the defeated Spanish Republic, who were fleeing from Francisco Franco's newly triumphant fascistic dictatorship. Despite much screaming and crying by the would-be boarders, the ship's captain strictly refused to allow anyone to board unless that person had a proper visa, thereby separating husbands from wives and parents from children.

That night, with the ship still moored in the harbor, small boats filled with those who were denied entry earlier in the day approached the ship. The Spaniards on board threw ladders over the side of the ship to the ones below. By daybreak the ship was filled to overflowing with those family members who had been denied earlier passage.

The Portuguese captain of the ship was greeted with a choice: take them all, or he would be put off the ship. Realizing that his captors had among them Spanish Admirals who could easily take his place behind the ship's wheel, the captain relented.

From the vantage point of their upper deck accommodations, the Revicis had an excellent view of the entire Casablancan harbor. The waterway was heavily populated with German ships and U-Boats. Dr. Revici once again took advantage of the situation and quietly took a series of pictures of the entire harbor with his camera.

Designed for perhaps 200 passengers, the crowded Portuguese ship now carried more than twice that number. Since the fascist government of Germany had supplied Franco's army in its overthrow of the Spanish Republican government, the wary passengers suspected that the German war ships and U-boats might begin to look for their ship as well. To protect themselves as they followed a zigzag pattern across the Atlantic, no lights were allowed on the ship at night. Although the ship's radio was kept on, they would not respond to any calls out of fear they might reveal their position to the Germans. During the transoceanic journey numerous calls regarding the whereabouts of their ship were left unanswered. As a result of the various precautions taken, the five-day journey took more than three weeks to complete.

Because of the severe overcrowding and the extended length of the trip, food and water were parceled. Despite the hardships, Dr. Revici reports that many of the passengers, glad to be alive, became "like brothers." Mantzi struck up close friendships with the chief surgeon of the Spanish Republican army along with other leading European physicians and scientists who were aboard. Although Dr. Revici no longer recalls discussing his research with the other passengers, it seems unlikely that he would have missed the opportunity.

As best as Nita can recall, the first long-awaited stop brought them to Havana, which was then under the protection of the British. After the British soldiers examined their passports, Dr. Revici handed over the snapshots he had taken earlier of the German ships occupying the Casablancan harbor. The Revicis didn't speak English, nor did the soldiers speak French. The soldiers acted disinterested, but two hours later the previous disinterest had been transformed into an invitation for him and his family to live in London—so pleased were the Britons with the marine reconnaissance photographs. After all the close calls and horrible events the Revicis had experienced in Europe, they were not nearly as excited by the offer as their prospective hosts were, so they declined.

The Revicis did take the opportunity while the ship was docked in Havana to wire the Merrys, who were by then located in the U.S., and who had tried unsuccessfully to contact the Quanza ship while it was at sea.

Besides having become the closest of friends with the Revici family, Gaston firmly believed in Revici's talents and wanted to help him in whatever way possible. The DuPont Corporation had offered Merry a position to act as the chief business representative for the entire South American operation for the DuPont paint company. But once Merry knew Dr. Revici had successfully escaped and would be relocating in Mexico City, he turned down the offer and indicated that he wished to work near Dr. Revici. DuPont complied with Gaston's wish and placed him in charge of their Central American operations. Despite the fact that the position was considered to be less prestigious than the South American assignment, Gaston gladly accepted.

Not only did Gaston and Nenette move to Mexico City, they took an apartment adjoining the Revici family. The two families knocked out the common wall between the two living quarters to create a huge two-family apartment. Because the Revicis had little or no money at that time, and Nenette's family was quite well-to-do, it is quite likely that the Merrys might have also taken care of the Revici family's monetary needs at first.

Soon after, with the help of E. Stoopen, M.D., a physician of both French and Mexican heritage, Gaston and Revici located a vacant hotel which they were able, with the assistance of Nenette's family money, to convert into a hospital. Nita would later describe Dr. Stoopen as, "probably the most darling man I've ever met in my life." Dr. Stoopen then joined Dr. Revici's research effort. Working alongside each other, the two physicians would also co-author several scientific studies.

With the help of the Merrys' money, the Instituto de Biologia Aplicada (IBA) was opened. Several of the highly qualified physicians whom Revici had met on the ship in their joint escape from Nazi-controlled Europe signed on almost immediately. "In two weeks we had a quality staff that would normally take ten years to bring together," Revici told me in an early interview. The chief of surgery for the Spanish Republican Army was one of those who would join Revici.

With the excellent staff and an animal laboratory, as well as an in-patient hospital, Revici was able to make important strides in the treatment of cancer and other conditions.

It was impossible to keep the positive results Revici achieved in cancer treatment a secret. Although Revici made no attempt to publicize his work except through the foreign medical literature, by 1943 word of his work spread to the U.S. The first major figure to contact him from there was a Wilmington, Delaware banker named Thomas E. Brittingham, Jr., whose father was one of the founders of the McArdle Memorial Laboratory for Cancer Research at the University of Wisconsin. Wilmington is also the corporate headquarters for DuPont, so it's quite likely that Gaston Merry or one of his associates had spread the word there, which then reached Brittingham. Through Brittingham, a number of top cancer physicians from across the U.S. would find their way to Revici's facility.

Although Dr. Revici had not promoted his research to the lay public in any way, patients also began to trickle in from various cancer centers in the U.S., particularly from those centers from where the visiting doctors had originated. The source of patients indicates that the visiting American doctors themselves probably spread the word among their own patients back home.

After three years of impressive successes with some of his cancer patients, the first attack on Revici's method appeared in the Journal of the American Medical Association (JAMA) in 1945. A disparaging letter, signed by some of the same doctors who had previously been impressed by Revici's work, was printed with a headline warning other physicians to avoid sending patients to Revici. Many more attacks were to come later. More will be said about the work done at the IBA in Mexico and the reactions of the U.S. medical establishment in Part IV of this book.

Before discussing those events it would be useful for the reader to have a working understanding in layman's terms of some of the many discoveries Revici has made. Those discoveries will be discussed in Part II.

Despite the initial salvo against Dr. Revici which appeared in JAMA, the following year Revici was invited to continue his research at the University of Chicago (UC) by Medical Department Chairman George Dick at the behest of Gustave Freeman, M.D., who had been a professor at UC prior to the war. Dr. Revici accepted the invitation. Unfortunately, within a week or two of Revici's arrival, Dr. Dick retired. Other parties at the university were not pleased to have Dr. Revici on staff, apparently due in part to the disparaging letter in JAMA. Another factor mentioned by Dr. Freeman was an escalating turf war experienced by many scientists returning from the war: "Sometimes a lab coat is used to hide one's dagger." As a result of those combined factors, Dr. Revici was never able to obtain hospital privileges at UC.

After a short time of being professionally stranded at UC, Revici turned down an offer to join the cancer research program at Illinois University and decided instead to move to New York City where he joined forces with the eminent urologist, Abraham Ravich, M.D. When Dr. Ravich was first introduced to Dr. Revici, he was in the process of obtaining a grant from the National Cancer Institute to study prostate cancer. Ravich became so impressed with Revici's work that he applied the entire grant to Dr. Revici's newly formed Institute of Applied Biology (IAB). Dr. Ravich would continue to support Revici's efforts over the years, continually donating money to the IAB until the two of them had a falling out over the use of Ravich's name in regards to a drug Revici developed that was marketed in Europe.

When Revici and Ravich first met, Ravich enjoyed a reputation that extended into the parlors of many notable and wealthy circles in New York. Ravich rubbed shoulders with federal court justices, a world renowned Catholic philosopher, and others. Despite his high social status, Ravich became Revici's main supporter and his right hand man when Revici established the IAB. Ravich used his connections to enlist Sara Churchill, the daughter of Sir Winston Churchill, to join the IAB board of trustees. Ravich was also instrumental in gathering much of the initial financial support for Revici's fledgling institute.

At the inception of the IAB, Ravich's son Robert, who was a physician in the Army, convinced the Army of the importance of Revici's research and was able to leave the post-World War II military to work with Revici. University of Chicago Professor Gustave Freeman also left the university and joined the Revici research team without pay for well over a year.

Through all the attacks made by organized medicine that would come over the ensuing years, a few individuals saw a different man. Professor Gerhard Schrauzer, an internationally recognized cancer researcher, told me in a telephone interview that he would place Revici's stature in medical history in the following manner:

> "There was Hippocrates, there was Galen, and then there was Paracelsus. He is among them."

Dr. Morris Mann, an independent physician-turned- inventor for numerous food and cosmetics companies, has studied steroids for twenty-five years. In a telephone interview, he said:

> Revici is 50 to 100 years ahead of his time in his knowledge of steroids. His work with steroids alone is earth shattering. I'm not fit to tie his shoelaces. In a hundred years people will say, "Isn't it a shame the way people treated Revici when he was alive?"

Some of Revici's patients have called him the Einstein of medicine or "another Albert Schweitzer." Albert Einstein himself is reported to have written Revici a personal letter after they met in the late 1940's.

The exact contents of the letter remain a mystery, however. It disappeared around the time a New York City fire marshal forced Revici to clean out a basement filled with papers. An overly enthusiastic group of volunteers carried out the task, and the letter vanished.

The second- and third-hand accounts of the contents of the letter are the stuff of legend. Before it disappeared, office receptionist Laura Whitney saw the letter and told Ruth Spector, an office volunteer, about it. According to Spector, Whitney said, "Einstein said Revici has the greatest mind he'd ever come across in his lifetime." According to Revici's own recollection, Einstein invited Revici to join forces with him on some other projects.

Whether the accounts of the letter have improved in the retelling is difficult to say. Certainly, a number of distinguished scientists and physicians who know him have said Dr. Revici is the most intelligent person they had ever met and a true genius. Did Einstein join that group? Possibly. Why would Einstein want to work in collaboration with Revici? And why didn't Revici take him up on the offer? Those are questions that could be batted around like sports talk around a water cooler, but accurate answers are difficult to come by. His niece says that Dr. Revici's personality won't allow him to work with anyone besides himself as the boss. It is true that Revici's fertile mind generates too many ideas to be constrained by other's input. Nita has said that when she worked in his lab, her father would show up almost daily with new ideas that he wanted to implement.

Whatever the contents of the letter might have been, Revici's primary focus has always been to develop medicines that could reverse cancer and other illnesses. This book will attempt to chronicle how successful he has been in those endeavors.

In Part II, we'll explore a number of Revici's more important discoveries and theories. I believe the reader will find them to consist of some of the most profound medical discoveries modern medicine has ever seen. Their fundamental nature is such that the answers to many illnesses and conditions could potentially be found.

In the case of a practicing physician, the truest test for any discovery or theory is to see how patients respond to the treatments. Part III will introduce quite a number of those patients. You might want to take a special note of the quality and vibrancy of life these patients experience and compare them with the experiences of cancer patients you have known. One certainty we all have is that all of us will die. A physician's task is to assist us while we are still alive to make our living years as healthy as possible—not just to keep us alive. As you meet the patients within these pages, I believe you will see that Revici has been successful in that area.

Unfortunately, Part IV of this book had to be written as well. In this world it seems that imperfections, shortcomings and even bad behavior are always with us. Dr. Revici saw glaring examples of those flaws before he fled Europe. As you will see, bad behavior is not limited to political dictators.

Part IV chronicles the major battles Revici has faced in his attempt to bring forward the best medicines he could. The Revici story is one of personal triumph and institutional tragedy. Part IV also tries to answer the question of how a cure for cancer could be hidden for so long.

Part V provides you, the reader, with some things you can do personally to help ensure that you can benefit from Revici's many contributions to mankind. This section will provide everything from ways to personally utilize some of Dr. Revici's findings, to how to get in contact with The Revici Life-Science Center for treatment. It also provides a plan of action for you to help make sure that Revici's medicines don't disappear into the dust bin of medical history.

So far, you learned a little bit about Dr. Revici's history. The next chapter will give you an idea of what it is like to be his patient.

2

My Dear, My Dear

Perhaps there is no better way to show the kind of
person Dr. Emanuel Revici is than to let Revici,
his friends and his patients tell it by way of an
oral history. What follows are stories told to
the author by some of the people who know him.

I knew a woman whose husband had left her with two small kids. She was so strapped, I would bring over food for her and the children. One of the children had asthma really bad, but her mother couldn't afford to take her to the doctor.

"So I went to Dr. Revici and explained the situation to him. He said to me, 'Please, please! Never talk to me about money. Bring me the child. I beg of you, bring me the child!'

"Well, the child started to get better, but she needed a certain kind of atomizer. So, Dr. Revici bought one for her and gave it to her mother.

"It wasn't until a few years later that I found out. Her mother men-

23

tioned it to me in passing because she thought I knew. Of course, Dr. Revici had never told me." *—Ruth Spector, office volunteer*

"You could call him at home any day, at any time. We called him three times on Christmas day including at 6:41 in the morning and 9:14 at night, plus at 6:30 in the evening on Christmas Eve. I kept a tab on all the calls we made. It totaled 437 calls." *—Pierce and Allan Hamilton*

"During all those hearings when they were trying to take his license away, they were so mean. Well, I went to all of them [the hearings]. The doctors on the panel never took any notes. When it came time for Dr. Revici to testify, he was advised not to tell them anything about what he did.

"His only response was, 'The world must know, the world must know.' When he started to speak, all the doctors on the panel started to write down everything he said.

"I talked to someone who worked in the governor's office about all the scribbling. He said that they knew Revici had the answer, and they were trying to get it.

"Then, during a later break, I was standing in a small hallway with Dr. Revici. By then I was furious with the whole panel and with what they were trying to do. I said to him, 'I hope they all get it [cancer] and have to come to you.' He looked at me and shrugged his shoulders. His lower lip came out. In disbelief, I said, 'You wouldn't!' He answered me with his soft, gentle voice: 'I'm 87. In all my life I've never refused to treat anyone. Would you want me to start now?'" *—Ruth Spector*

"Dr. Revici was the person who treated my first wife when she died of cancer in 1969.

"I've always been appreciative of what he did for her during the daily telephone calls to Jamaica, West Indies, where she died. After her death I again visited his office, this time to offer him a $5,000 check to cover his phone calls and other expenses, but, again, he was adamant in his refusal." *—Lyle Stuart, publisher, Barricade Books*

Revici told the following story on himself: "When I first started practicing I never charged. But some of the patients told me they couldn't come to see me because of it. So I had to charge them, so they could get care."
—Dr. Emanuel Revici

"Dr. Revici was offered an enticing opportunity to practice medicine in a Middle Eastern country to treat the royal family and other important people. Revici told those who invited him that if he were to go there, he would have to be able to treat all patients, not just selected people. When that condition wouldn't be met, Dr. Revici turned down the offer."
—Marcus Cohen

"A child who had been treated by Revici became hospitalized in Atlanta with a severe case of asthma. For two weeks the little girl failed to respond to the medical treatment given her by the hospital physicians. The mother decided to call Dr. Revici at home. He had given the mother his home number as he does with all his patients. It was midnight.

"He answered on the first ring. He suggested a treatment over the phone and told her to call her back. The mother had already accumulated a number of Revici's different medicines, so she was able to treat her daughter herself, even though she was in the hospital. She ended up calling Revici back at two in the morning and at three. He was awake for all the calls. By morning the woman's daughter had recovered and was able to be discharged."
—Ruth Spector

"When Dr. Revici was running Trafalgar Hospital in New York, they had a problem with getting some of the patients to take their medicine. The treatments were totally free to the patients with all the expenses paid for by donations from wealthy benefactors. To get the patients to use the medicine they had to start charging them five dollars. It worked."
—Lawrence LeShan, Ph.D.

"Even Revici had limits to his patience. A woman came to him who was close to death. She had cancer throughout her body. Her doctors pre-

25

dicted she would die within two or three months. Her recovery under Revici was swift and dramatic. She never returned to her other doctors.

"Three months later one of her original physicians called her home to see if she was still alive. When she answered the phone, the doctor asked about his patient. He didn't recognize the perky, energetic voice on the line. When the doctor had last seen her, the patient barely had enough energy to speak, breathily uttering one word at a time as if each word might be her last. When the doctor finally realized he was speaking to his former patient he exclaimed that he must meet Dr. Revici.

"But when Revici was informed of the other doctor's response, Revici refused to see him, 'I will never see this man after what he did to you! He should have known after the third x-ray.' The doctor had apparently used the patient like a lab animal, x-raying her repeatedly. He didn't want to teach his method to someone who didn't value human life and human dignity.

"Ten years later the woman was handling multi-million dollar loan contracts for Fanny Mae. Revici has never seen the doctor."

— Ruth Spector

"Once when Dr. Revici was in London, there was a machine that could apparently measure alpha, beta, gamma and delta brain waves. He was hooked up to the machine. According to the tester, Revici's brain waves were complete in both hemispheres for all of the different brain waves, something that had previously only been seen with certain Eastern mystics." *—Alice Ladas, Ed.D., author*

"Dr. Revici heard about a patient who was too sick to come and see him. He paid the man a house call, walking up five flights of stairs. Revici was ninety-three." *—Marcus Cohen*

"This being New York, we had a kind of boast in the hospital that made it different from any other hospital: every patient would be spoken to in his own language, which in New York doesn't happen all the time.

"One day a Japanese priest came in, and he didn't speak a word of English. We knew damn well, although he speaks six languages, Revici didn't speak any Japanese. So, that morning everyone went on rounds to see how he would handle it. The son of a [gun] did the examination in Latin. It must have been the first time a physical exam was done in Latin in a thousand years." *—Lawrence LeShan, Ph.D.*

"The patient was bedridden with AIDS, and his condition was considered terminal. A friend called to see how he was. The woman who answered the phone said, 'I'm sorry, he's gone.' The caller asked when he had died. She answered, 'He's not dead. He went shopping.' The patient had begun treatment with Revici one week earlier."

—Norman Carmen

"We had a conversation with a couple outside the office. They were both members of Mensa, the club for people with extremely high I.Q.'s. They said Dr. Revici had taken the test, but his score was too high to be accurately measured." *—Allan Hamilton*

"After hearing my mother wasn't doing well, Dr. Revici made a home visit. He spent two hours. On the second visit he spent the entire night. About three or four in the morning I saw him up. My mother died three or four days later. I felt a special closeness with Dr. Revici, but I believe he treated all his patients that way. I have a special warm feeling even now for Dr. Revici." *—William Rosenberg*

"One time I was in the office and was sitting next to a gentleman, a young fellow. I struck up a conversation with him. To this day I can still see that guy. He said, 'You know, no one has ever given me anything in this life. Nobody has ever done anything for me.' What happened to him is, he had cancer of the lung. He went to see Revici. He was out of a job. Revici said he would take care of him. He would treat him. 'So, I told him I didn't have any money.' Revici said, 'That's all right, I'll still take care of you.' I can still hear that guy. He was sitting there, and he was like, 'Nobody, *nobody* has ever done anything for me.' He couldn't believe that this man was going to do something for him. It just tore me up inside listening to his story." *—Allan Hamilton*

"There were never two minutes when the phone didn't ring right through dinner. We expected it and understood."

—*Nita Taskier, Revici's daughter*

"He always said 'My dear. My dear.'" —*Pierce Hamilton*

"There was a patient who had a front room in the hospital with a telephone and a window with a view of some trees. After eight months, she ran out of money to pay the hospital bill. That meant she would have to go on state assistance and would have to be moved to the ward. She was upset by the prospect. I went to Dr. Revici and told him of the patient's concern. Revici said he would see what he could do, and sure enough, she was able to stay in the front room until she died four months later.

"After her death, I quietly looked into it to see what had been done. That's when I found out that Dr. Revici had quietly paid the difference in the woman's bill so that she could stay in the front room with her telephone and her view of the trees." —*Lawrence LeShan, Ph.D.*

"During the eighties, the office was under a lot of financial pressure due to a number of law suits and the resulting lawyers' fees. We were in danger of having the electricity and the water cut off. Dr. Revici hadn't received any salary for years.

"It was during this time that he came out to the receptionist, who also collected payments from patients. He told her, 'I don't want to know who pays, and who doesn't. I don't want it to affect my treatment.'" —*Ruth Spector*

"I talked to a doctor who was performing his own research on Revici's method after hours at Sloan-Kettering. He told me it showed very promising results. As Revici's lawyer, I told the doctor that we would need him to testify in Revici's behalf. When he refused, I told him we would have to subpoena him.

"The doctor burst into tears and begged me not to make him do that. He said he had a family, and that he could lose everything when the people at Sloan-Kettering found out about it. The doctor was beside himself. I told him I really needed for him to come forward, not so much to testify regarding the results but to testify about the punitive climate that existed at the hospital regarding anything to do with Revici. Although the doctor begged not to be dragged into the case, it was my duty as Dr. Revici's attorney to let my client know about the other doctor. The doctor's testimony had the potential to show clearly that Dr. Revici's method was not being given fair consideration by the mainstream medical community.

"Dr. Revici decided not to have the doctor subpoenaed. He didn't want to risk the other man's professional future—even if it was to his own benefit."   —*Sam A. Abady, attorney at law*

"When Dr. Revici would read my charts, he was like a wise old turtle. He would submerge himself in the chart, sinking bit by bit. After a long while he'd slowly come up from the depths."   —*Meade Andrews*

"I'd written down a phone number on a slip of paper while talking to someone on the phone. Dr. Revici was in the room at the time of the conversation. A couple days later I wanted to call the person back, but I couldn't find the paper I'd written the number on. He became aware of my frustration. He asked me to wait a minute, and then he closed his eyes and went into what looked like deep thought. After about two minutes, he recalled the number. He was in his late eighties or early nineties at the time."   —*A. R. Salman, M.D.*

"My mother had developed a severe, chronic angina. She had gotten it when we had to make a terrifying, two-mile run through a wooded no-man's-land to escape the Nazi soldiers who were patrolling the area. Her condition became so bad after six months that just raising her arm would bring on an attack. She was completely bedridden and at risk of having a heart attack.

"My father was very concerned. He said he didn't know what to do, because he had developed a medicine that might work for her, but due to the circumstances we found ourselves in, he hadn't been able to test it for safety. We told him he didn't have anything to lose, because she would surely die if something weren't done soon.

"So, he gave her an injection, and then another. Two days later she was up and around. Within a week or so, she was able to go out shopping." [Author's note: She lived another 24 years]   —*Nita Taskier*

"He was like the finest European gentleman."   —*Charlotte Louise*

HIS DISCOVERIES

3

Pain and Cancer:
A Major Clue to Curing It

*"Genius is seeing what everyone else sees and thinking what
no one else thinks. Revici is a genius."*

ROBERT FISHBEIN, M.D.

Revici didn't find instant success in his quest to solve the puzzle of why the pregnant Romanian woman's terminal cancer disappeared. Instead, Revici's early research with human placental extracts administered to humans produced contradictory results. On some occasions patients injected with the extracts showed a remarkable reduction in pain. In a few cases the pain would disappear entirely for hours. After a few treatments the pain would sometimes disappear for days.

With other patients, however, the pain would almost immediately intensify and would sometimes become unbearable. To make matters worse, some of the patients who had previously benefited in the short term would, after continued treatment, begin to experience a new pain which became more severe as the treatment progressed. Yet, he surmised that he might be on to something, because he was usually eliciting a dramatic response, even if it wasn't always in the right direction.

Moreover, with a few patients, remarkable and long-lasting results were achieved. One case concerned a fifty-six-year-old man with a nasty tumor that involved more than half his tongue. "The mouth lesion was very painful and bled," Revici reported in his 772-page book, *Research in Physiopathology As [A] Basis Of Guided Chemotherapy With Special Application to Cancer* published in 1961. With injections of the placental extract the patient's condition improved rapidly. Within two weeks the tumor started to shrink. But by the fifth week, treatment had to be stopped due to increasing pain. Yet, despite the cessation of treatment, the tumor continued to shrink. Patient follow-up continued as well, "...for another year-and-a-half, during which time there was no recurrence. After that the patient left town, and we were unable to reestablish contact with him."

In another case a woman, "...came under our care with a massive tumor filling the entire vagina." A biopsy eight months earlier indicated a Grade III cancer, which meant that her chance for a cure was nil. By the time she began treatment with Revici her tumor, "was protruding from the vagina as a hard mass." With the placental treatment the patient improved and her pain was, "entirely controlled within a week." Treatment continued for a total of forty-five days, when it was interrupted. She returned after three months. An exam revealed that her tumor had entirely disappeared. Her case was then followed for two years with no recurrence of the cancer.

But for the most part long-term success was elusive. Such contradictory results perplexed Revici and beckoned him to go to Paris to study the matter further unencumbered by his private practice and professorial duties.

A major part of the solution came from an unexpected direction. In those early years patients with cancer received only limited amounts of narcotics for pain relief. This meant that the natural ebb and flow of any pain the patient experienced was not entirely masked by the effects of medication.

Like many of Revici's discoveries, his finding would come about from a simple observation that had gone unnoticed by others. Revici observed something about that ebb and flow of his patients' pain, and he would call his discovery "dualism," which meant that cancer patients have either one of two possible, opposite pain patterns.

Revici observed that some cancer patients woke up in the morning with very bad pain which would diminish in the late afternoon and evening. Other cancer patients woke up without that intense, early-morning pain, but as the day progressed into the afternoon and evening, their pain grew progressively worse. Revici theorized that the cause of the different pain patterns might correspond to an overly acidic (low pH) or an overly alkaline (high pH) level, as measured at the site of the tumor.

Revici's hypothesis was supported by additional observations. He found that patients with morning pain were provided some measure of relief by eating. Patients who experienced most of their pain in the second half of the day found that eating would intensify the level of their pain. The observed increase or decrease in pain occurred regardless of the tumor's distance from the digestive system.

Since eating usually causes a temporary shift towards alkalinity in the blood, the possibility that alkaline pain would be made worse by eating made sense. It also made sense that eating would help lessen, to a temporary degree at least, the pain of acid pattern cancer patients. According to Revici's scientific text previously mentioned, patient behavior appeared to support Revici's observations, "many whose pain was increased with the intake of food refused to eat for fear of aggravating their suffering, while those of the other group wanted to eat whenever pain was severe in order to reduce its intensity."

Revici decided to conduct some studies of his observations to see if there was a connection between urinary pH levels and cancer pain.

Revici first established that healthy people have an average urine pH of 6.2, although it fluctuates throughout the day. Specifically, healthy people have a pH urine cycle with readings above 6.2 beginning around 4 a.m. each day This cycle continues for approximately twelve hours. At approximately 4 P.M. the pH shifts to readings below 6.2 and continues to remain above 6.2 until approximately 4 A.M. the next morning.

The next step was to compare the pH readings of healthy people with the pH readings of cancer patients. Revici kept track of the urine pH of the patients on an hourly basis. Meanwhile, he asked his patients to keep track of their average pain intensity during each hour. The results were highly significant both in the pH readings and in the pain registered by the patients. The pH readings of the patients were stuck.

Some patients had pH readings that were always stuck above 6.2. But other patients were always stuck below 6.2. Only rarely, if ever, did most of the patients show a reading that crossed the 6.2 line.

The pain cycles of the patients also corresponded to the aberrant readings. Patients who had lost the alkaline part of their cycle (4 A.M. to 4 P.M.) experienced much greater pain in the morning and early afternoon than they did in the evening. Because those patients were stuck in an acid cycle, Dr. Revici labeled this phenomenon as an acid pain pattern.

In contrast to the first group, the patients who had lost the acid part of their pH cycle (4 P.M. to 4 A.M.) experienced much more severe pain during the late afternoon and the evening hours. Because those patients were stuck in an alkaline cycle, that pattern was labeled as an alkaline pain pattern.

In either case, more pain was experienced when the patient went into the abnormal phase of his or her pH cycle. The pain was usually at its worst when the aberration was greatest. In numerous cases, charts showed patients whose pH never crossed over to the opposite side of 6.2 for a period of fifty consecutive days. In those patients the worsening of pain consistently corresponded to the daily 12-hour period when the patients failed to manifest the appropriate pH cycle. As Dr. Revici wrote in his book:

> In many of these patients, variations in pain intensity could be seen to follow a pattern. Although the variations are usually referred to as "spontaneous", we could show that they were related to the time of day....In one group, pain was severe in the morn-

ing and diminished toward evening, while in another group, little or no pain was felt in the morning and exacerbations occurred in the evening.

Furthermore, the patients who were sickest from a clinical standpoint had the most extreme imbalances, with constant pH readings that were consistently either far higher or far lower than 6.2. It did not make any difference whether the extreme readings were always alkaline or always acid. From the pH charts, Revici noticed that the severity of a patient's conditions appeared to correlate with the severity of the imbalance as shown in the patient's chart. As patients' physical conditions worsened, their pH scores would become more aberrant.

Those many connections demonstrate that the abnormal pH readings were not just an artifact of the patient's overall condition, they were part and parcel of the illness itself.

Those studies also indicate that a dualism exists in cancer, that is cancer could exist when a malfunction occurs in either the acid pH cycle or the alkaline pH cycle of a patient. Therefore, it was logical for Revici to conclude that a successful treatment for cancer would be one where the patient's urine pH fluctuated normally from alkaline to acid each day.

Revici conducted similar tests for pain patterns among cancer patients with other biochemical markers which he would also demonstrate to be connected to the condition of cancer. For example, increased levels of potassium in the blood serum were associated with increased pain patterns.

Revici decided to see if he could affect the pain levels of cancer patients by treating them orally with various acid and alkaline solutions. Once again, pain was dramatically, if temporarily affected. Acid solutions temporarily reduced or eliminated alkaline pain patterns. Alkaline solutions did the same to acid pain patterns. On occasion, when alkaline substances were given to patients showing alkaline pain patterns, the pain increased. Similar aggravating responses occurred by giving acid solutions to patients with acid pain patterns.

The next step for Revici was to see what type of response would occur if the acid and alkaline compounds were applied directly to tumors. In his previous tests on animals, normal tissue was relatively unaffected by the various compounds, while tumorous lesions reacted much more dramatically. Now Revici was ready to see if the results he achieved with lab animals would also occur with humans.

"Patients with easily accessible superficial lesions, especially tumors, in which painful areas could be well localized…" were chosen as subjects for this experiment, according to Revici. They would again keep hourly records of pain intensity. Meanwhile, Revici devised special equipment and procedures to isolate and measure the pH levels of the exposed tumors.

As expected, Revici found the pH of cancerous tissue to change with the application of the different substances. The patients experienced dramatic drops in the intensity of pain which corresponded to the changes in pH. It is also interesting to note that non-cancerous tissue on the same patients showed very little or no change in the surface pH when the tissue was subjected to the same acidic or alkaline substances. The results of that testing provides further evidence that the source of the disturbance in urine pH comes from the aberrant pH of the tumor itself.

In a few cases, an alkaline compound was placed on an alkaline tumor. Typically, the pain would increase so dramatically that the experiment would have to be quickly reversed by introducing an acidic compound. The same type of experiment was done with acidic tumors with similar aggravation of pain.

More pH studies were performed on patients with other pathological conditions and symptoms during those early years in Paris. He found similar correlations of dualism in a number of conditions, such as asthma, some types of vertigo, some types of hearing loss and manic-depressive disorders. One of the most interesting examples of dualism was the symptom of itching.

Very little is understood about the cause of certain types of itching such as is found with pruritis. Itching can result from any number of causes, such as insect bites, an external irritant or a disease state. In testing dualism, Revici found externally caused itching did not have a dualistic characteristic. In contrast, he found that itching resulting from a pathological condition often did have the same dualistic feature as some of the other illnesses he had examined. Like the other dualistic conditions, the severity of the itching displayed a close correlation to the severity of the imbalance. As Revici continued his research over the next six decades, he would find numerous conditions whose pathology exhibited either a dualistic pattern or a single sided pattern of pH imbalance.

Revici found that some conditions always produce an alkaline pain pattern reaction. One example of such a condition is any trauma that damages tissue, such as broken bones, burns or surgery. The finding that surgery produces an alkaline pattern reaction would play a large part in informing Revici as to why surgery might cause a patient with alkaline pattern cancer to react to surgery with a rapid regrowth of the tumor, or with the seemingly spontaneous appearance of metastases. Even today, decades after Revici's findings, that sequence of events occurs all too frequently.

For example, baseball legend Mickey Mantle was treated for liver cancer by surgical means. His liver was removed and replaced with a healthy one. Although it wasn't immediately reported to the public, the surgeons had to leave behind a small piece of the tumor.

Within a couple weeks a virulent cancer had invaded his lungs. According to the Washington Post, one of his doctors, Daniel DeMarco M.D., reported that he'd never seen a cancer spread so fast, "[T]his was the fastest, most aggressive tumor we've ever seen." Apparently ignorant of Revici's widely disregarded findings, first made as early as 1930, Mantle's doctors expressed the hope that Mickey Mantle's fame would help to make organ donations and transplant surgery more popular. Based on their continued advocacy of liver transplants, it can be assumed that his doctors never considered the possibility that the surgery itself may have contributed to the virulence of Mantle's tumor.

Revici made his finding regarding the effect of surgery on the spread of cancer 65 years ago and discussed it in his book in 1961. Despite Revici's early warning that coincided with the height of Mantle's playing days with the New York Yankees, the widespread practice of surgery continues unabated even today. The reappearance of cancer, either in the same place as the previous surgery or elsewhere is often responded to with shrugs, as if it were just bad luck rather than as a direct result of the surgically induced alkaline imbalance. As of this writing, the medical profession still hasn't accepted the possible role of surgery in promoting the growth of cancerous conditions.

Also unrecognized is the possibility that any major surgery can lay the groundwork for future cancer by aggravating an alkaline condition in a patient who might already be tending towards that pattern of imbalance. This is not to say that every surgery produces cancer, but based on Revici's findings, it might be a good idea to evaluate a patient's acid/alkaline pattern for a few days before subjecting them to the knife.

Revici's observation regarding the impact of surgery on the acid/alkaline balance of the patient helps to explain why surgery is a risky treatment for many cancer patients, especially when the physician is unaware of the patient's pH pattern. Surgery isn't necessarily a good idea for acid pattern patients either in that it's difficult to predict the extent of the alkaline reaction that the surgery will cause.

There are limited circumstances where Revici believes surgery might be indicated, such as localized, easily accessible tumors with no metastases, for a patient with an acid pattern. In the vast majority of cases, however, surgery is a higher risk option than previously understood, particularly in the hands of physicians unaware of the alkaline effects of the surgery they perform.

Radiation is another alkaline-producing procedure. Typically, patients who undergo radiation and have an acid pain pattern will show short-term progress followed by a reversal and the downward spiral of the patient's condition. In contrast, the condition of patients with alkaline pain patterns will worsen immediately after a radiation session. Because radiation is often directed to the site of the tumor which might be alkaline, the radiation can very well aggravate the response in surrounding tissue. This could result in a rapid spread of the malignancy or an activation of undiscovered metastases. Since pH levels are not generally considered by radiologists, the patient can suffer in either case.

Revici's finding of dualism in cancer and other pathologies was just the beginning of his many important medical discoveries. The next step was to find a way to move cancer patients out of the pattern in which they appeared to be stuck. If acid pattern patients reacted positively to alkaline compounds, then the solution might have appeared to be to give those patients some of those alkaline substances until they recovered. Alkaline pattern patients could likewise be given some acid substance to affect a cure.

Of course almost nothing is that simple when it comes to the workings of the human body and of cancer in particular. Substances given either orally or by injection often go through a series of chemical changes in the body. This can result in little of the original substance reaching the site where it is needed, while increasing the potential for the medication or its byproducts to cause new problems. A way had to be found to effectively deliver medications that could change the acid/alkaline patterns of patients without harming them. In the next chapter we'll see how a class of substances called lipids came into play.

4

More Than Just Blowing Bubbles

"I am pleased to learn that his [Revici's]
concept of surface tension in biology bore fruit..."

GUSTAVE FREEMAN, M.D.

Like many of Revici's discoveries, his ability to develop a method for effectively delivering medications in cancer cases resulted from converting a simple observation into a series of important scientific advances. Revici noticed, like a lot of people had noticed, that tumors were rather impervious to the effects of their environment. The relative stability of tumors is in marked contrast to the multitude of fast reactions taking place thousands of times a second in the human body.

Many different chemical reactions are occurring in the human body all the time. Different body salts combine with various compounds constantly. Proteins and amino acids also regroup constantly, and carbohydrates quickly break down into simple sugars. With each of those changes the characteristics of the new products can be quite different from the previous ones. One common characteristic for most of those reactions is their water solubility.

Revici theorized that rapid, water-soluble reactions played a much lesser role in cancer metabolism because tumors don't change much in character from one moment to the next. He theorized that there must be a substance that would provide the stability tumors manifest. That idea of a stable, non-water soluble substance led him to look at lipids as a likely place to find some answers. He wrote, "They form a group 'apart' from all the water-soluble constituents, a fact which permits them to function without continuous interference from the other constituents."

In his early research he found placentas to be extremely rich in certain kinds of lipids. Yet, as we already know, the placental lipids had a wide-ranging, unpredictable effect on tumors. Sometimes they helped, and sometimes they made the cancer worse. When they did help, oftentimes the benefit was short-lived, only to be followed by a reversal and deterioration of the patient's condition.

In his 1961 book Revici reports that in over one hundred cases of terminal cancer treated with placental extracts at various hospitals in Paris between 1935 and 1938, objective improvement was seen in only 20% of the cases. By objective improvement he meant that the tumors of the patient had measurably shrunk or disappeared. The percentage, although low, was not so bad considering that other doctors sometimes sought him out to treat their most seriously ill cancer patients. In addition, the dramatic, short-term positive results led him to believe he had found a part of the answer. However, a 20% objective response rate still meant there was much room for improvement.

By 1938 Revici noted that the placental treatments often produced a permanent shift into alkaline pain patterns among patients who previously had suffered from acid pain patterns. In addition, patients who had already been diagnosed with alkaline pain patterns experienced a marked increase in pain when treated with placental medications.

As he continued his search, Revici combed the scientific literature on lipids only to find them to be a largely ignored topic to the point that even the definition of what comprised a lipid was inadequate. Striking out largely into unexplored territory, he learned through his own research that some lipids would promote an acid reaction in the urinary pH while others promoted an alkaline reaction. That finding would become one of the most important discoveries he would make in the treatment of cancer and other dualistic diseases. With that finding Revici had found a way to attack cancer, whether it exhibited an acid imbalance or an alkaline imbalance.

With this new information, Revici decided to drop placental lipids as a treatment due to their overly alkaline properties that were often difficult to reverse, and replaced them with two categories of lipids with antagonistic properties: fatty acids and sterols. Revici found alkaline pain patterns could be controlled with the highly unsaturated fatty acid lipids almost immediately, while the sterol lipids did the same for acid pain patterns. "In both cases, the effect occurred in a few minutes." Tumor shrinkage would often follow within a matter of days or weeks.

At first the choice of medication was determined solely by the patient's pain pattern. By 1938 Revici was monitoring the patient's urinary pH as well. He also began to monitor the specific gravity of the urine, urinary calcium and the total blood potassium. Revici found that sterols and fatty acids had many different properties including opposite effects on urinary specific gravity, urinary calcium and blood potassium.

For example, he found that he could use the results from tests on urinary calcium and total blood potassium to isolate imbalances at the cytoplasmic level. (Cytoplasm is the material that surrounds the nucleus of each cell.) For conditions affecting the extracellular compartment, blood serum and lymph, he found that he could isolate imbalances by applying a dualistic interpretation on urinary pH, urinary surface tension, pain patterns and blood eosinophiles (a type of white blood cell.) To detect imbalances occurring at the organ level, application of the dualistic principles in interpreting urinary specific gravity and body temperature proved effective.

Some critics have faulted Revici's use of specific gravity by pointing out that the specific gravity of urine is greatly affected by the amount

45

of water in the urine. What those critics have failed to note is that Revici devised a way to take the water concentration into account by using a mathematical index which eliminates the effect of the fluctuation caused by the water content of the urine sample.

The ability to isolate imbalances through their alkaline/acid characteristics as well as at the particular level of their biological organization would prove to be quite useful.

Although he had chemical agents to attack both acid and alkaline tumors as early as the late 1930's, he encountered a problem with most of his patients in that during the course of treatment their lab results would switch to the opposite side. That is, acid pain patterns would switch to alkaline pain patterns, with their corresponding lab results, and vice versa. Although treatment would be stopped, the patient would sometimes continue to get worse and would often die. Revici included two cases in his book that date back to the 1930's that illustrate the challenge.

In one case a patient bedridden with cancer in both his lungs recovered quickly. After less than two months of treatment with fatty acids, the sixty-six-year-old man went horseback riding. He continued the same treatment for two more months until the condition took a sudden turn for the worse. Two weeks later he would die from an accumulation of fluid in his lungs.

A sixty-eight-year-old woman fared better. Her Grade IV breast cancer—the worst of four staging categories—had attacked the bones of her legs, hips, ribs, spine and skull. These types of cases are the bane of cancer medicine because little can be done except to try, most often quite unsuccessfully, to decrease the patient's pain. Yet, with the application of the proper lipids in this case, the woman's pain gradually lessened and disappeared. Within five months all of the patient's bones had healed, and she was discharged from the hospital. After no treatment for more than two years, she was examined again. According to Revici, she showed no signs of her previous condition, and, "[s]ubsequently, because of the war [World War II], I lost contact with her."

The above case is merely an anecdotal account, if one is inclined to lean in that direction. Yet it is an anecdotal account with enough chemical changes to make numerous bones solid while causing the tumors to disappear—thus it could be said that it is a good anecdotal account. Good anecdotal accounts have been the basis for the discoveries made by such great scientists as Pasteur, Fleming, Semmelweis and many others. The ability to ignore a good anecdotal account is a key trait of the mediocre scientist.

With the ability to monitor pH levels, specific gravity and other indicators, Revici started to modify the choice of lipids used based on the patient's lab tests. It is not clear from the record when Revici first began to switch from one type of lipid to its opposite when a patient's lab results switched. The first case history where he mentions doing so occurred in 1942, in Mexico. It's quite likely that the switching technique took place much earlier, however, because of his ability to monitor specific gravity by 1938 and urinary pH earlier still.

The 1942 case provides a dramatic example of the success obtained by monitoring and switching, nonetheless. In her seventies, a nearly comatose woman's deeply sallow skin color made her a poor candidate for survival. She had a stomach tumor and a liver tumor which reached all the way down to her groin area. After more than a month of steady improvement from the treatment, she took a sudden turn for the worse. Revici wrote, "Analysis at this time showed the opposite off-balance present." At that time her treatment was changed, and she continued to improve once again. Her liver, once ballooned beyond belief, was back to normal size within one year. She died nine years later, at the age of 83, of a heart attack.

This adjusting back and forth to his patients' "off-balance" was implemented time and time again. By monitoring the patients and changing the medicine accordingly, good results often followed. Revici's individualized approach towards treatment was a novelty at the time and flew directly in the face of the strict cookie cutter regimens that had become "de rigeur" at that time and that have only recently seen any modification. While conventional medicine saw his approach as one of chasing after placebo effects, Revici saw conventional medicine's adherence to strict regimens as unscientific.

Another related approach that proved effective was to give a combination of different fatty acids to patients with an alkaline imbalance and a combination of sterols to patients with an acid imbalance.

For example, there was the case of a woman with a Grade III abdominal cancer. Two tumors, eight inches in diameter, "gave her distended abdomen a very irregular appearance," Revici reported. After three weeks of treatment with the sterol of cholesterol, no improvement was seen. Her medication was changed to glycerol, another sterol. Another three weeks passed without any noticeable improvement. At that time both the cholesterol and the glycerol were administered together. The combination brought rapid results. Within a month the obvious abdominal tumors were no longer evident to the touch. A noncancerous ovarian cyst was located and removed surgically. At the time of the surgery only white patches were found where the tumors had lain before. "There were no recurrences during several years of follow-up, after which we lost track of the patient," Revici wrote.

For reasons that will be explained in a later chapter, the above approach of using multiple lipids often produced beneficial results where a single medicine had not.

When Revici received the annual medal from the Society for the Promotion of International Relations on November 13, 1961, he presented a lecture touching on the highlights of his discoveries. In that speech he told of the results achieved with one of his patients. The example is worth rendering almost in its entirety here because it demonstrates the direct relationship between the application of treatment of the off-balance and the improvement of the patient:

> "We first saw a patient, Mrs. M. B., in a terminal stage with a tumor of the ovary and multiple metastases in the liver, spleen, intestine and [the abdominal lining] as revealed by an exploratory [surgery]. Biopsy proved it to be an adeno-carcinoma. Our analysis indicated an off-balance requiring agents with a negative polar group. The result of their administration was good. The massive tumors disappeared and the patient resumed a normal, active life.
>
> "Unaware of her condition, and against our advice, she stopped the treatment. Two years later there was a recurrence of the con-

dition. A [large tumor below her diaphragm] and a large tumor in her lower abdomen brought her rapidly to a pre-terminal stage. A biopsy was performed and revealed the same tumor. In view of the good results obtained the first time, treatment was started again with the same agents, in spite of the fact that the analysis now showed an opposite off-balance present. The immediate result however was totally unfavorable subjectively and objectively. We changed consequently to the opposite agents, with a positive polar group this time, as indicated by the analysis. The condition was once again well controlled, the new masses disappearing, and the patient once more resuming a normal life.

"Still unaware of her condition, the patient continued the treatment—but at very irregular intervals. Within a few months a new mass was found in her abdomen. Once more [an exploratory surgery] was performed showing again an inoperable tumor. A biopsy obtained from a nearby gland indicated the same tumor.

"The analysis now indicated an off-balance opposite to the second one, that is, similar to that seen the first time. With the administration of the corresponding agents, the mass disappeared. At this time the patient was informed of her condition, and she continued her treatment without interruption. Now, six years later after her last recurrence and eleven years since we first saw her, she is in perfect health.

"We present this case because it shows clearly how important it is to consider the specific off-balance in order to ensure the selection of the proper agents. Incidentally, we also want to emphasize the direct relationship between treatment and the results obtained. *The fact that, in this patient, the condition evolved three times and each time was controlled only when the adequate treatment was instituted, excludes the possibility of repeated spontaneous remissions.*

"*In hundreds of cases, the correlation between treatment and the results obtained has been as direct as in the case presented above.* Many of our patients with different tumors originating in almost all the organs, are now clinically free of tumors, living normal lives years after their condition had been considered hopeless....

"Pre-terminal or even terminal cases are now seen to respond better, that is, more often, more rapidly and more completely with subjective and objective favorable changes....

"In spite of all the interesting results already obtained, we still look upon our approach as being in its beginning, especially in its application in therapy.... Over and beyond the specific results which have stemmed from this approach, we put it forth here with considerable confidence as opening the way to an entire field of further research in clinical science in particular and in basic science in general." (emphasis added).

By the time of his lecture in London, Revici had developed 30 different ways to identify either an acid or an alkaline pattern in cancer patients, including several lab tests he devised on his own. One of the most interesting was his invention of a device he named the "Urotensiometer" to measure urinary surface tension. He earned a patent for the glass tube device, the design of which was dependent on a complex mathematical equation. Revici began using the Urotensiometer at least as early as 1948. By the time Revici's book was published, he had conducted more than 100,000 lab tests using the device to monitor the progress of patients.

Ironically, present day medical science is of the opinion that there is almost no role in biology for surface tension. The one major exception to that belief is based on a discovery by John Clements, M.D., concerning the lung development of pre-born infants. Dr. Clements has earned international recognition for his pioneering work in that area.

Assisted by a team headed by Julius Comroe of the Cardiorespiratory Institute at the University of California in San Francisco, Dr. Clements isolated and identified the lipid responsible for maintaining the proper surface tension on the surface of pre-born babies' lungs. Today, through amniocentesis, physicians can determine the lung development of the pre-born child, thanks to Dr. Clements.

Determination of lung surface tension is also used to alert physicians of potential lung abnormalities. As a result of his work, Clements was awarded the annual prize for research by the Trudeau Society and was given an honorary professorship at the University of Berne, Switzerland.

Dr. Clements' discovery came from a good anecdote. He had become intrigued with the "blowing of bubbles," that he noticed on the alveolar surfaces of infant lungs. (The alveoli are the miniature balloon-like surfaces of the lungs where oxygen mixes with the blood.) He later told a former associate that he had wondered if surface tension might have something to do with the formation of those bubbles.

The former associate was Gustave Freeman, M.D. It was Dr. Freeman who had previously mentioned to Clements the possibility that surface tension might have some application in biology. Clements would later tell Freeman that it was his suggestion that caused him to come up with his hypothesis regarding surface tension in regards to bubbles. Freeman's source for the possible role of surface tension in biology came directly from Revici during the time that they had worked together in Chicago and New York. In a letter to me, Dr. Freeman wrote, "I am pleased to learn that his [Revici's] concept of surface tension in biology bore fruit..."

Clement's important discovery was made without any awareness by the medical community that its genesis came from Revici.

By isolating and identifying a lipid to be the cause of lung surface tension in infants, Clements confirmed one of the fundamental tenets of Dr. Revici's work regarding the role of lipids in biology. Revici has long held that acidic lipids increase local surface tension on the outer surfaces of cells and in the blood, while alkaline lipids decrease local surface tension in the same areas. The alveolar surfaces of the lungs would just be one example of an outer surface of cells where Revici would expect surface tension to play an important role.

From the early days of the mid-1930's up to today, Revici has continued to refine and improve his use and understanding of lipids. He was the first to propose that lipids act as a "lipidic defense system" which functions separately from the immune system, but which protects the body from viruses, bacteria, funguses, cancer and a host of other diseases and conditions.

One of his major breakthroughs with lipids, which began in the 1950's and has continued ever since, has allowed him to incorporate elements like selenium, copper, sulfur, or zinc into the lipids, thereby making the lipid bases an efficient carrier of potent substances, transporting them exactly to where they are needed. This advancement will be discussed in a later chapter.

Another breakthrough in Revici's design of medicines has enabled him to send the most potent forms of medicine to a tumor site. This potent discovery which he calls "twin formations" is used to describe a special type of connection between atoms. His incorporation of minerals into lipid carriers and his twin formation discoveries are monumental advances in medical treatment. Both will be discussed more fully later on.

But first to more fully appreciate some of these discoveries, you'll first want to go on a guided tour of Revici's revolutionary theory of evolution that goes beyond Darwin and radically changes the presently held hypothesis of evolutionary genetics. With this knowledge it will be easy to see how Revici has flung the doors of medicine wide open in a way that will dramatically alter the approach to conquering viral and bacterial infections in addition to numerous other diseases.

5

Cancer, AIDS, the Ebola Virus and How Life Was Formed

"And yet, it moves!"

GALILEO, IN ANSWER TO CHURCH CRITICS
WHO INSISTED THAT THE SUN REVOLVED AROUND THE EARTH,
AND WHO WERE ABOUT TO CONVICT HIM OF HERESY IF HE DIDN'T RECANT.

One week after his ninety-eighth birthday, Revici said something in his soft Romanian-French-German-Italian-Spanish accent that was similar to Galileo's famous remark. He spoke slowly with a lilt that gave each phrase the opportunity to sink into this listener's ears: "How much longer will I live? One year, two years, maybe five? At my age I could die any night. It does not matter. What happens to me is unimportant. What I have discovered, I *recognized*. I didn't make it up; it is a fact. It may take five years, ten, twenty or maybe even more [for others to recognize these discoveries], but it is a fact."

Although Revici probably wasn't thinking about Galileo when he made those remarks, it is worthwhile to briefly recount the history of Galileo's ordeal here because of the ways it ties into Revici's own story.

Within a hundred years or so after Jesus of Nazareth walked the earth, a Greek astronomer and geographer named Ptolemy drew some maps that supposedly laid out the respective paths that each of the then-known planets traversed. The charts showed our very own planet at the center of the universe with the sun revolving around our earth. Ptolemy's argument hinged on an amalgam of circles only an astronomer could love. But its defenders clung to it as if the existence of God hung in the balance.

Today we know Ptolemy was quite wrong, yet his theories held sway for 1,500 years.

Galileo contended that the earth circumscribed the sun rather than the other way around. Even though he had more than enough evidence to prove his point, he had trouble convincing many of those in high places. On occasion he needed to flee from his persecutors, and was placed under house arrest for a number of years. Left with little choice, he finally pretended to agree with his tormentors in order to save his own life. Yet Galileo's response under his breath at his trial told those close to him— and ultimately the world—that he knew the truth would not change, regardless of his plea or the self-righteous attitudes of his foes.

Today it might be difficult to understand how supporters of Ptolemy's theory could have been so unyielding in their opposition to Galileo in the face of so much evidence to the contrary. Yet, as you read this book, you will see that although the years change, the willingness by some to look askance at the most overwhelming evidence has not.

In one respect Ptolemy's chart is a bit like the mysterious periodic table of chemical elements many of us learned to hate in high-school chemistry. The periodic table, which frequently appears as a large wall chart, is made up of squares almost as confusing as Ptolemy's circles.

The good news is that, unlike Ptolemy's circles of his universe, the periodic table is an accurate depiction of the chemical elements and provides us with useful information. However, the information it provides is still somewhat limited. Revici's additions bring the chart to life.

The difference between the old chart and Revici's might be likened to the difference between reading the music to Handel's Messiah and hearing it sung by the Mormon Tabernacle Choir. While the former is useful in a limited way, the latter certainly has its advantages.

Although the finer points of Revici's approach to the periodic table are best understood by experts, Revici said it would take a person who is strong in chemistry "two weeks" to learn the basic principles behind his theory. Just as we don't have to be music experts to enjoy *The Messiah*, the rudimentary aspects of Revici's enhancements to the periodic table can be appreciated by almost anyone.

On a practical level, Revici's enhancements offer researchers a blueprint into the formation of all life. Part of Revici's approach, which he calls "Hierarchic Organization," acts as a support system for his startling theory of evolution. Revici's theory of Hierarchic Organization provides a road map into the workings of every level of life, from viruses on up to humans. As a former senior medical scientist of Johnson and Johnson, the late Arnold Cronk, M.D., once told Benjamin Payn, Ph.D., "Revici is a fountain of ideas that could keep an entire graduating medical class busy for the rest of their lives."

It is important to note something about Revici's theory. No theory is any better than its practical application—Ptolemy proved that. So when one examines Revici's theories, it is useful to keep in mind that he has tested them in his laboratory and demonstrated their validity by making patients well.

He spent 74 years, both in clinical practice and in the laboratory, testing and fine-tuning his ideas. Unlike Ptolemy, who did not even have a telescope, Revici has based his findings in the lab on tens of thousands of animals and applied the results to thousands of patients.

Furthermore, his theories and applications have received recognition, if not in the United States, then from prominent international organizations. For example, the aforementioned Society for Promoting International Scientific Relations, which included 14 members who would be honored with the Nobel Prize, awarded Dr. Revici its annual medal in response to the publication of his book in 1961. The award was a confirmation of the validity of his theories by some of the most upper-echelon members of the international scientific community.

Unfortunately, his book can be difficult to read—even for physicians, many of whom are not trained in physical chemistry and atomic physics. Prior to publication of Revici's book, his niece's husband, then a senior editor at the University of Chicago Press, cautioned Revici that his book would have difficulty finding acceptance in the United States due to its unusual ideas and his manner of presenting them.

Any discussion of Revici's theory of Hierarchic Organization can easily become an extremely complex affair, fit only for the rarefied air of those who are at home in a multitude of scientific disciplines. Revici supports his arguments by relying on quantum physics, electromagnetic fields and van der Waal's cohesion forces, etc. to explain in precise, technical language *why* certain steps in evolution were able to take place. This chapter will focus on what took place in plain language. It is possible to highlight in layman's terms a few of the basic aspects of Hierarchic Organization as Revici uses it to explain the connections between chemistry, biology, evolution and medicine.

It all starts with evolution.

Let's first consider the prevailing evolutionary theory, which is that all life came from the sea. Revici forcefully argues that the theory of all life coming from the sea is quite wrong. Revici contends that life started on land—specifically, in the mud—and migrated to the sea before returning to the land once again.

At first blush the argument over whether the precursors to human life started in the mud or in sea water might appear to be arcane and of little significance to the practice of medicine. As the reader shall soon see, however, understanding the difference is essential for the proper application of medicine.

For example, a correct understanding of the fundamental building blocks of human evolution provides a great advantage in treating a multitude of health problems. Just as a good mechanic needs to know the proper order in which to reassemble an automobile engine, physicians and their patients would benefit immensely from a proper understanding of how the human body was first put together. Revici knows how to repair the human engine because he knows how it is formed.

Revici's evolutionary theory is based in part on the premise that any evolving life would need to have an abundant supply of whatever elements it needed to ensure its short- and long-term survival. To test his theory, Revici decided to look at the human cell to see what is actually in it. He wanted to compare the ingredients of cells to what was available on the land, in the air and in the ocean.

He found a heavy concentration of carbon and nitrogen inside the nucleus of cells. Both nitrogen and carbon are much more heavily concentrated in the atmosphere and in the earth's crust than they are in the ocean. The two elements were probably in abundant supply due to the relatively frequent volcanic action that occurred in the early part of the earth's existence. Furthermore, those two elements can readily combine into a nitrogen-carbon-nitrogen-carbon (N-C-N-C) formation, according to Revici. This formation, when combined with hydrogen, produces a strong positive electrical charge, which makes it conducive to attracting formations with negative electrical charges. Sure enough, the N-C-N-C formations are the basis for numerous amino acids and nitrogenous bases found in the nucleus. (Amino acids and nitrogenous bases are both important compounds for the formation of proteins, which are important building blocks for life.) These findings provided tenuous but useful support for his ideas.

More convincing evidence comes from examining the fluid layer outside the nucleus of cells which is referred to either as intracellular fluid or cytoplasm. Revici took note of the fact that the concentration of potassium is 59 times higher in the human cytoplasm than is found just outside the human cell (extracellularly). He also noticed that this ratio is quite similar to the concentration of potassium in the earth's crust compared to that found in the ocean. In fact, the concentration of potassium is 61 times higher in the earth's crust than it is in the world's oceans. The two ratios of 59:1 and 61:1 are close enough to each other to be considered a match.

Revici also compared sodium and potassium concentrations in the blood serum. For example, the concentration of sodium in human blood serum is 16 times higher than is the concentration of potassium in the extracellular human blood serum. Not so coincidentally, the Pacific Ocean's sodium concentration is 16 times higher than its potassium concentration.

It should be noted that sodium and potassium are almost inter-changeable in chemical reactions—that is, they will combine with the same elements, if given the chance. The most common examples of that fact being sodium chloride and potassium chloride, both table salts. This means that if both elements had been available in equal abundance both on land and in the ocean, it is highly unlikely that the large ratios given above would exist in intra- and extracellular development.

If the ratio of intracellular potassium to extracellular potassium is approximately 60 to 1, and the ratio of the earth's potassium to that of the ocean's is also approximately 60 to 1, then the evidence suggests that the cytoplasm was formed on land.

If the ratio of sodium to potassium in the ocean is 16 to 1, and a 16 to 1 ratio of sodium to potassium exists in our extracellular compart-ment, then the evidence suggests that the extracellular compartment evolved in the ocean.

Because the lipid layer of the cytoplasmic level acts to keep out the material of the extracellular level, it is clear that the development of the cytoplasmic layer preceded the formation of the extracellular level.*

Thus, Revici hypothesized that the intracellular formation of life took place on the earth's crust prior to the formation of the extracellu-lar component which took place in the ocean.

For an independent perspective on the extracellular fluid, it is worth considering the words of Sherwin B. Nuland, M.D., who teaches surgery and the history of medicine at Yale. In his magnificent book, *How We Die* he discusses the extracellular fluid:

> It is as though the earliest groups of prehistoric cells, when they first
> began to form complex organisms in the marine depths from which
> they drew sustenance, brought some of the sea into and around
> themselves so that they might continue to be nourished by it.

---

* For reasons that are far too complex to try to explain here (van der Waal's cohesion forces, etc.), the positive electrical charge of the N-C-N-C-H played a role in the formation of the subnuclear and nuclear compartments, which preceded formation of the cytoplasm.

To get a picture of how this evolutionary process worked in human development, picture a type of nucleus that was hanging out in the mud for a period of, say, a few billion years. There was an abundance of potassium around. According to Revici, some of those nuclei found the potassium to be quite useful, so they incorporated it, not into the nucleus, but as part of a new surrounding layer which we call the cytoplasm. The nucleus already had a membrane which prevented much of the potassium from penetrating it. Therefore, the potassium compound was taken up by the cytoplasm outside the nucleus. (To protect the cytoplasm, a lipidic layer came into play as well, but I'll discuss that more later in this chapter.)

In the course of a billion more years, some of these new life forms, with their cytoplasmic coats, migrated successfully to the sea. These cells found an abundance of sodium in the sea. But the sodium was unable to penetrate the lipid protection surrounding the cytoplasm. Yet, over a period of many millions of years, the life form successfully incorporated the sodium into its lifestyle, outside the cellular membrane—or as Dr. Nuland wrote, "brought some of the sea into and around themselves so that they might continue to be nourished by it." Again, a lipid protection was added in order to keep the sodium concentration intact.

Thus, we can see that the potassium-rich layer came first, thereby forming the intracellular layer, while the sodium-rich layer came next and formed the outer layer. The lipid-rich coating around the intracellular layer provided the insulation that kept the potassium and the sodium apart, thereby keeping the ratios intact.

A few more years went by, relatively speaking, and some of the cells with the potassium undercoat and the sodium overcoat migrated back to dry land. Because lots of time had passed, the old neighborhood had changed quite a bit. Meanwhile, the plants that stayed behind for those many millions of years had done their part by making free oxygen available in abundance. This enabled the returning life forms to do things they had not been able to do before–like develop lungs.

Some of the sodium-coated creatures remained in the sea and developed along their own evolutionary path without lungs. With the exception of a few marine mammals that need to come above the water to breathe, aquatic life has followed a lungless evolutionary path. That is, the development of lungs is exceedingly difficult unless there is an abundance of free oxygen, as is found in the atmosphere.

The terrestrial plant kingdom was also unable to utilize the oxygen because it lacked the capacity for generating the appropriate extracellular surface tension. It is widely known that one of the major differences between plants and humans is that plants have only a potassium rich intracellular fluid but they don't have the sodium rich extracellular lipid compartment. Because plants didn't go through the critical stage of adding the sodium coat and its additional layer of lipid protection, they are unable to provide the necessary surface tension to utilize oxygen despite its relative abundance on land.

If we recall Dr. Clement's discovery discussed in the previous chapter regarding surface tension and lung development in prenatal infants, it would appear that Clement's findings fit quite nicely into Revici's evolutionary theory.

One of the main features of Revici's evolutionary theory is that it proposes a layered approach to evolution. That is, simple life became more complex by slowly adding discrete layers to itself to create whole new entities. An essential factor in the ability of lower life forms to keep adding layers to itself is the series of lipid-rich compartments that were formed. Without those compartments a chemical change would be far less permanent. For example, the potassium rich cytoplasm of an organism would have eventually been replaced with sodium molecules once the creature migrated to the sea. Therefore, the lipid layers provided the stability needed to keep a species intact.

To see another way in which Revici's evolutionary theory is different from conventional wisdom, let's consider the present widely held theory of evolution by looking at the lowly virus.

The present thinking on evolution is that one day, one of the viruses had a stress put on it that was so great that it went through a genetic mutation, making it possible for a particular virus to reproduce a different entity. From that day on, it was capable of producing a new life form. Over time these mutating occurrences resulted in the life forms of various bacteria. Thus, new life forms were made by genetically branching off from their viral ancestors. As these great stresses continued, they caused more genetic changes which, in turn, produced funguses and other life forms. Continuing over a period of eons, the process produced all the plants and animals and humans that exist today.

Revici disagrees with that scenario. While Revici's ideas and those more generally accepted on evolution are only theories, the differences are important. Revici's theory has enabled him to make discoveries and effective treatments for diseases which he could not have made had he held on to the more popular evolutionary theory.

Revici says that viruses came about as a result of proteins that have added a layer of nucleic acids. He views the proteins of the virus as the primary layer and the nucleic acid as the secondary layer. He points out that viruses possess an interesting feature due to the simplicity of their structure. A virus that appears to be inactive and thought to be dead can come back to life if it is given a new nucleic acid. Revici sees the virus as being at the same organizational level as the genes or possibly at the level below genes.

Let's look at Revici's theory of the virus's evolutionary role in the formation of bacteria. Revici argues that a bacterium is composed of a virus that has attached itself to nucleoproteins and fatty acids.*

As it turns out, each bacterium contains a protein and a nucleic acid, which are the primary and secondary parts of a virus, and an added layer of nucleoproteins combined with fatty acids. The fatty acids provide the lipid envelope that stabilizes the secondary layer of a bacterium.

According to Revici's argument, viruses came into an environment rich in nucleoproteins and fatty acids which, under the right circumstances, allowed them to generate the new level of life forms we know as bacteria. Revici states in his book that bacterial organisms are at the same organizational level as the nuclei for reasons that are beyond the scope of this book.

---

* Different bacteria may have different acid secondary parts, such as the thio-organic acids or other special acids. Different strains of bacteria may also have genetically different viruses as their primary part.

This is not to say viruses don't mutate genetically. It says that when viruses do mutate genetically, they remain viruses, and that mutation within a species is a separate branch of evolution. Through genetic mutation a number of different viruses can be produced, but a virus can never produce anything but a virus in this manner. Revici's theory says that a virus doesn't genetically mutate to become a different type of life form, but adds a new layer of nucleoproteins and fatty acids to do so and thus becomes a bacterium.

In the hundreds of millions or even billions of years that it may have taken for the successful merging of primary and secondary layers to produce bacteria from viruses (and fungi from bacteria etc.), genetic mutation certainly occurred along a non-parallel track, thereby resulting in many different kinds of viruses. It is this genetic variety that accounts for the variety of different bacteria, fungi and other life forms. It is important to note, however, that without the addition of the material of the secondary layers, not a single bacterium, fungus or other higher life form would have ever been formed, according to Revici.

There is a simple yet profound question that arises from Revici's theory of the evolution of a virus merging with a secondary material to produce bacterial microbes. Why doesn't the virus eat the bacterium? It turns out that the answer to that question has in it the answer to AIDS, the Ebola virus and every other viral infection that concerns modern man.

Revici reasoned that the answer had to be simple. For a bacterium to be a viable life form, despite its viral interior, it must have a natural defense that protects itself from the noxious aspects of its viral core. Without that natural defense, the virus would consume the microbe. Bacteria's defense, Revici reasoned, had to be contained within the secondary part of the bacterial organism.

Because fatty acids and nucleoproteins are the main constituents that make up the secondary layer of bacterial microbes, it was likely that at least one of those two compounds would provide the natural defense that protects the viability of a bacterium from its own viral aspect.

Revici has solved the above question in a way that helps to confirm his evolutionary theory and has enabled him to develop a series of anti-viral drugs in the process.

In an experiment performed on rabbits, Revici tested a number of substances, including fatty acids and nucleoproteins, for their anti-viral properties. The fatty acids proved to be entirely resistant to viruses. The experiment demonstrated that the natural defense mechanism with which bacteria protect themselves comes from the fatty-acid lipids, which also happen to be one of the lipid categories Revici uses to treat cancer. Revici also found that fatty acids combined with nucleoproteins have an enhanced anti-viral activity.

In the same study, Revici determined that viruses respond to sterols and fatty alcohols in the opposite manner. Both sterols and fatty alcohols feed the virus and accelerate viral replication. According to Revici, sterols are lipids that are antagonists of fatty acids. Fatty alcohols are a category of compounds with lipidic properties that are also antagonists of fatty acids.

Further support for Revici's Hierarchic Organization comes from the relationship of fungi to bacteria. According to Revici fungi are the next step up the evolutionary ladder from bacteria. Therefore, any fungus should have a natural defense in its secondary layer against its bacterial core. As Revici points out, many anti-bacterial agents are made from fungi. That fact lends support to the idea that each fungus has a natural defense which protects itself from the noxious effects of its bacterial core, and this is further evidence supporting Revici's theory of a layered evolutionary world.

As you will recall, Revici had theorized that lipids are stable compounds within the body due to their lack of solubility in water. That non-solubility would be an important feature if a substance were required to provide a constant layer of protection from an organism's primary layer. Revici then theorized that there must be a lipidic layer at every succeeding layer of evolution. He decided to call this series of layers the "lipidic defense system" due to the apparent ability of lipids to defend a life form from the noxious organisms contained within itself. (At levels below the nuclear, the defense mechanism appears to be electromagnetic rather than lipidic, according to Revici.)

Another important aspect of his theory is the natural layer of protection each lipidic level provides, which acts as a form of insulation to separate itself from the level above it. As we've seen from the discussion on potassium and sodium, that insulation allows each level to act somewhat independently from the other.

The lipidic defense system acts loosely like our system of roads. We have interstate superhighways for traveling from one state to another (system). The state highways can get us from one city to another (organs). Major thoroughfares get us in and out of the city (tissues). Busy streets take us around the neighborhood (cells). Side streets take us home (nucleus). Our driveways give us somewhere to park (subnuclear). There is a connection between each system of roads, but they tend to operate separately.

With the knowledge that each layer functions somewhat independently, a whole new approach to medicine is possible. By determining the secondary part of a particular layer, it becomes possible to intervene in an illness at whichever layer a condition is occurring, as was done with fatty acids against viruses. In his book, Revici published his findings regarding the dualistic effects of lipids applied to different layers of the evolutionary chain, including viruses, bacteria, protozoa and complex organisms. Those findings still remain a treasure yet to be discovered by researchers and the medical profession.

The examples of the virus-bacteria-fungus chain has direct application to human biology. Revici considers viruses to be "at the same level as genes or even the level below genes". Bacteria are at the same organizational level as the nucleus, according to Revici, while single-celled organisms, such as fungi, correspond to the human cell level.

Whether or not each human cell has a virus-like entity as one of its building blocks, remains to be seen. The implications of that very real possibility are far-reaching, indeed.

If bacteria correspond to the nucleus of the human cell, it has grave implications for any anti-bacterial medicine that doesn't take into account Revici's theory of Hierarchic Organization and may explain, in part, why anti-bacterial medicines that are generally available have side effects.

One way to view Revici's lipidic medicines is to liken them to putting a loose tiger back into its cage where it can do no harm. Standard medicine shoots any tiger that is loose, but leaves the gate open for more tigers to escape. Today's medicine might also end up shooting a lot of innocent tigers still in their cages in its attempt to stop the loose one. In the human body our bacterial "tigers" are essential to our health. Thus, killing them with antibiotics may sometimes be ill-advised.

We might define biology as living chemistry because what else is an organism but a bringing together of chemicals with life breathed into it? If biology is living chemistry, then it follows that biological functions must comply with the same principles as chemistry does. Yet the complexity of those two fields has made the search for their seminal connections an elusive quest.

Revici's premise is that just as biology is a series of layers of chemical compounds separated by lipids, a similar pattern might be found in the layers of electrons found in chemical elements (see appendix B).

In high school chemistry it is taught that each chemical element has one or more electron rings which surround the nucleus of the atom. The periodic chart of chemical elements reflects the number of electron rings a chemical element has by its horizontal position on the chart.

Specifically, the top horizontal row of the chart is reserved for those elements with only one ring. The second row of the chart is for elements with two electron rings. The third row of the chart is for elements with three electron rings, and so on for each of the seven rows.

With more rings an element has room for more electrons. The number of electrons an element has is determined by the number of protons the atom has in its nucleus, because it is the positive charge of the protons that holds the negative electrons in the atom's orbit.

Revici's premise is that each of the horizontal rows corresponds to a biological compartment. As you shall see, the elements from the lowest, or seventh horizontal row, correspond to the lowest level of biological organization while the elements from the top, or first row, correspond to the most complex level according to Revici. A comparison between potassium and sodium provides a useful example once again.

As stated earlier in this chapter, Revici found that potassium corresponded to the intracellular, or cytoplasmic, layer in biological organization. As you will also recall, potassium is much more heavily concentrated in the earth's crust than it is in the ocean. When looking at a periodic table, one finds potassium on the fourth row from the top, the same horizontal row as calcium, iron, copper, nickel, chromium, zinc, selenium, bromine, titanium, vanadium and manganese. All of those elements are also most heavily concentrated in the earth's crust.

Furthermore, the elements of the fourth horizontal row are found in heavier concentrations in the cytoplasm than those of the third horizontal row of the chart. Not so coincidentallly, the third horizontal row is filled with elements that are found in heavier concentrations in the ocean than the elements in the fourth row.

A similar correspondence is seen in the human organism. The elements of the third horizontal row of the periodic table are also more concentrated in the extracellular compartment of the human organism than the elements of the fourth row of the chart.

Moving up the chart we find a similar situation. The air is almost entirely comprised of elements from the second row of the periodic chart. Revici sees a correspondence between the second row of the chart and the development of the next level of biological complexity beyond the extracellular compartment.

From those observations Revici surmised that the top horizontal row of the periodic chart could correspond to the development of the systemic level of the human organism. The second level of the periodic chart corresponds to our organs, including the lungs. The third row of elements corresponds to what Revici calls the metazoic level and includes the extracellular compartment, the blood serum and the lymph.

The fourth row corresponds to the intracellular compartment otherwise known as the cytoplasm. The fifth row of elements corresponds to the biological nuclear compartment. The sixth horizontal row of the elements corresponds to the subnuclear compartment according to Revici. The seventh row, which contains the radioactive elements, corresponds to the primitive level. Revici proposes that the radioactive component of the seventh level elements might possibly be the physical source for life.

To test his hypothesis of Hierarchic Organization, Revici administered small but toxic amounts of either rubidium, potassium or sodium to mice. To track the injected material, radioactive tracers were used.

He found that rubidium, which is found on the fifth row of the periodic chart—the row Revici associates with a cell's nucleus—typically caused an abnormal fluid space limited to the nucleus of the mice's cells.

Potassium, an element from the fourth row of the chart—the row Revici associated with the cytoplasm—caused the same type of damage as the rubidium, but it was limited to the cytoplasm.

When the mice were injected with sodium, which is found on the third row, the row Revici associates with the extracellular area, the only damage was found in the extracellular area.

The experiment would indicate that Revici's premise regarding a correspondence between the periodic chart and Hierarchic Organization is correct. With that correspondence he found two direct medical applications for his findings. Because the elements seem to gravitate to the level of biological organization that corresponds to its evolutionary development, Revici found that such information could be used to better interpret the results of lab tests.

From his knowledge of lipids Revici understood that each lipidic layer had the effect of causing each biological compartment to work somewhat independently from the others. For Revici, knowing in which layer of an organism an element is most heavily concentrated has enabled him to treat various illnesses with pinpoint accuracy.

For example, Revici knew from his experience that patients who were stuck in an acid off-balance pattern often exhibited a deficiency of potassium in their blood serum. Revici's knowledge that the blood serum wasn't the controlling compartment for potassium in the cell led him to examine what was happening with those patients' potassium levels at the cytoplasmic level. Through laboratory analysis he was able to differentiate whether a patient suffered from a general potassium deficiency, or if the problem resulted from excess use of potassium in the patient's cytoplasm.

Thus, a correct understanding of the potassium readings often provided Revici with the necessary information needed to correct the root cause of the problem for the betterment of the patient. Without that knowledge a physician might incorrectly prescribe an increase in a patient's potassium intake which would not correct the excess utilization problem and might actually intensify the patient's condition.

A second way that Revici has been able to use his knowledge of the correspondence between the periodic table and biology was to target certain elements to a patient's condition. First, Revici would determine the compartmental level of a patient's illness, which he typically did through various tests and clinical observation.

With the proper diagnosis, including the compartmental source of the illness, he would tailor the medications to include the appropriate elements needed by the patient. In a later chapter the reader will see how large doses of individual elements such as zinc, copper, calcium, selenium or potassium are targeted to the needed compartment without causing toxicity.

Revici's compartmental theory of Hierarchic Organization works in conjunction with another concept. As you will recall, Revici identified a condition he called dualism in a number of illnesses where either of two opposite conditions could cause the same illness. In the last chapter we saw cases of cancer accompanied by either an acid or an alkaline off-balance. In humans the alkaline cycle breaks body constituents down, while the acid cycle builds them up. Both processes are necessary for health. This process of tearing down is more commonly known as a *catabolic* activity while the building up process is called an *anabolic* activity.

As Revici further explored the periodic table of chemical elements, he noted another interesting fact. The elements in each particular vertical column were either all catabolic in their behavior or all anabolic.*

For example, the first vertical column is comprised of the elements hydrogen, lithium, sodium, potassium, rubidium, cesium and francium. All of those elements are anabolic. The second vertical column contains beryllium, magnesium, calcium, strontium, barium and radium. Each of those elements in the second column are catabolic. Revici

---

* The lanthanides and actinides series are exceptions to this pattern for reasons that are beyond the scope of this book.

has used his knowledge of the catabolic/anabolic characteristics of the individual elements to enhance the effects of many of the medicines he has developed.

In atomic physics there is a similar dual process of anabolism and catabolism. One is a magnetic force that pulls the electrons in toward the center of the atom. The other is an outward force that pushes the electrons out. Together the two countervailing forces keep the electrons of each atom in their particular orbit.

Chemists and physicists call the two forces *electromagnetic* and *quantum* forces. With only the electromagnetic force, all the electrons would just smash together like a huge, very tightly compacted ball of aluminum foil. Revici termed that force to be an anabolic force.

On the other hand, if the only force in existence were the quantum force, electrons would fly out of their orbit away from the core of the atom. If a quantum force were allowed to act without opposition, it would cause objects to break into many smaller pieces. The quantum force is considered to be a catabolic force by Revici.

If either extreme of anabolism or catabolism were to occur unopposed in the human body on a grand scale, we would either implode or explode. Obviously that doesn't happen.

But what if either the anabolic or the catabolic force happened on a very small scale to a relative degree? What if, in a localized area of our body, there was a preponderance of anabolic, build-up energy? Or, alternately, what if, in the same spot, we had too much catabolic, tear-apart energy? We might not be dead, but would it make us sick, and would it cause pain?

In terms of chemistry, what if the configuration of an atom or a compound became "lopsided" energetically due to a minute imbalance in the structure? Would it affect the function of the atom and those around it? If biology is living chemistry, would a slight energetic imbalance in the chemical structure of an element or compound have the potential to make a person sick?

All of the above is an oversimplification of what Revici hypothesized and, most importantly, found answers to. He then asked more questions and probed more deeply into the ramifications of Hierarchic

Organization and was rewarded with some fascinating answers. Those answers have the potential to shake the foundation of what we know about nature and the world.

The word "foundation" is often overused to describe the effect of one thing or another, and this author pleads guilty to using it rather freely in this book. One proper use of the word is to denote the foundation of a house. Everyone knows that when the foundation of a house shifts, it affects more than the basement of the house. If the bottom of the house shifts, the whole house is at risk.

Consider if a shingle flies off the roof of a house. In that particular case we have an isolated problem which, in the short term, will probably turn into a worse problem only if it rains or snows. But there will be no shift in the house because, unlike a foundation, a shingle bears none of the structure's fundamental properties.

Revici's insight into the building blocks of life is comparable to a house's foundation. If one of the lipidic compartments begins to function poorly, it is relatively easy to see that any number of physical problems are likely to result. It should be equally easy to see that the repair of an improperly functioning lipid would also have the effect of correcting many different physical maladies.

Consider that without the lipid compartments there would be no single-cell animals, nor would there be any of the more complex living creatures from the invertebrates all the way up to the human form. Understanding the fundamental importance of lipids at almost every layer of life helps us to appreciate why Revici's work has such an enormous impact on medicine.

One advantage of Revici's principles is that once a research scientist, chemist or physician learns the theory, he or she can begin to make remarkably accurate predictions about the effects of each element and its resulting compounds—both in the laboratory and on patients. In short, Revici's theory is a scientist's dream—a discovery road map.

When more scientists are exposed to Revici's principles of Hierarchic Organization and Dualism, the likelihood of an explosion in discoveries is greatly increased. Physician and inventor, Dr. Morris Mann, is a good example of that possibility. Dr. Mann makes a good living as an independent inventor, creating new cosmetic and consumer products for major companies. If his inventions didn't work, he would be without an income, so he relies on the most advanced knowledge of chemistry available to give him an edge.

Dr. Mann has written that he and his colleagues have found Revici's approach to be, "a major contributor to our understanding of structure/function relationships in pharmacology." Dr. Mann also considers Revici's contributions in medicine to be great enough to put him in the same company as Sir Alexander Fleming, the British physician who discovered penicillin.

Another physician, Dr. Lynn August, has said of Revici's discoveries and theories, "I saw his book, and a thousand lights went on. It's part of how I think." Among other findings, Dr. August has found that the common affliction of premenstrual syndrome (PMS) has both anabolic and catabolic forms. With that discovery she has been able to treat both types successfully.

So, in addition to his individual discoveries, it appears that Revici has opened windows into the discovery process. If the responses of Drs. Mann and August are any indication of the effect Revici's book could have on science and medicine, it means that the scientific community would be able to accelerate its search for the answers to today's medical mysteries like never before.

Yet, four months prior to the official release of his book, Revici, like Galileo, failed to convince his critics. His acceptance by the international scientific community was effectively nullified by the American Cancer Society (ACS) in the United States. In a publication earmarked for professionals in the cancer field, the ACS printed an op-ed article of less than three hundred words entitled "Unproven Methods" about Dr. Revici and the Revici Method.*

Largely as a result of the targeted ACS piece, Revici's book sat unread in the publisher's warehouse. Revici has often said, "The

---

* Advance copies of Revici's book were circulated in the scientific community, including the American Cancer Society. Mention of Revici's book was conspicuous by its absence in the brief ACS article.

American Cancer Society burned my book," an allusion to the Nazis' treatment of disapproved books and from whose clutches Revici had escaped twenty years earlier.

Had the American Cancer Society or the American Medical Association looked at his work and recognized its value, this book would not have needed to be written. Meanwhile, his facts are gnawing at the medical establishment's foundation. And like Galileo's planet earth—it moves.

6

The Difference between
a Dade Man and a Dead Man

"Other than that, Mrs. Lincoln, how did you like the play?"

Many of the people who disapproved of Galileo's theory of the earth circling the sun were not familiar with the science of astronomy.

Likewise, most physicians in the U.S. and elsewhere are not trained in the specialized field of physical chemistry. That shortcoming may help to explain why some physicians are baffled by much of Revici's work. Physical chemistry considers what effects the structure of a chemical compound has on its functions.

For a better understanding of how structure can determine function, a few examples outside the field of chemistry might be useful. Consider the following hypothetical newspaper headlines:

Driver Brakes Car	Driver Breaks Car
Boy Sits on Elephant	Elephant Sits on Boy
Dade County Man Honored	Dead County Man Honored

In each of the above examples, each pair of headlines contains exactly the same letters within the pair. Although the letters are the same, the order of placement of the letters is slightly different. Yet the slight change of structure has a dramatic effect on the meaning of each headline.

We have obvious examples in our own anatomical structure. For example, shoulders have a different range of motion than elbows. Those differences are determined by the different design of the two ends of the upper arm bone. If that bone were installed in reverse, the function of our arm would be dramatically different from what it is now.

In chemistry differences in the structure of identical elements can also result in dramatic differences in function. The most striking example of structure affecting a molecule is probably exhibited by the differences between the soft, opaque graphite in a pencil and the incredibly hard, clear structure of a diamond. The two items are chemically identical except for their structures. Both are made from pure carbon, but graphite carbons are linked in a simple chain pattern while diamonds are more pyramidally structured, with the pyramids alternately pointing up and down.

Graphite and diamonds are not the only examples of structural differences within identical chemicals. Revici has taken advantage of the effects of structural differences within chemical compounds in a number of different ways.

For example, in the early 1940's he studied the effects of radiation on the lipidic defense system of rats and noticed a very important event. The irradiated rats physiologically responded to the radiation by changing slightly the molecular shape of a fatty acid. This minor change in shape nevertheless caused a large quantity of an abnormally structured fatty acid to be produced. By using the technique of spectral analysis, Revici found one of the carbon atoms in the fatty acid compound had rotated from its proper position. The change in structure of the fatty acid was the same as that found in cancer when the cancer was associated with a fatty acid abnormality.

Through further research Revici determined that the minor change of positioning in the carbon atom caused the fatty acids to lose their ability to latch onto oxygen molecules. In his experiments with rats, the loss of oxygen produced a localized rancid condition. The rancidity would then worsen until the animal died.

The minor rotation of an atom on a molecule became so critical to the life of the rats, that Revici found he could predict their deaths by performing a chemical test. He devised a complex chemical reaction that allowed him to measure the concentration of oxalic acid present in the fatty acid. He found all the irradiated rats would die when the concentration of oxalic acid reached an index of fourteen to seventeen, but they would usually not die before then. The oxalic index also provided confirmation that it was the amount of abnormal fatty acids that caused the death of the rat. Revici has also found that an oxalic index on humans can provide an important measure of the state of health of patients.

To treat the abnormal fatty acid produced in the rats, he relied once again on the importance of structure to determine function. He knew from previous work that a fatty acid antagonist would provide the best antidote. By testing various fatty acid antagonists, he settled on the fatty alcohol known as butanol. There are four butanols, each with a different structure and a different effect. One had no effect, two had a limited effect, and the fourth, n-butanol, provided the best effect due to its particular structure.

Since that time Revici has demonstrated the healing effects of n-butanol for radiation burns. That finding has proved to be particularly useful, especially in cases where radiation treatments have resulted in overdoses and burns. Fifty years after Revici's ground-breaking research, there is no FDA approved medication that is as effective as n-butanol in overcoming the deleterious effects of radiation treatments and burns.

Revici's discoveries for the treatment of radiation burns and radiation shock were deemed to be so important that twice the U.S. Navy attempted to recruit him for top-secret work regarding the U.S.

nuclear weapons program. All the more impressive is the fact that Dr. Revici was not even a U.S. citizen at the time. The first time they made inquiries, he was still a resident of Mexico. Revici turned down both offers, however, due to his consuming interest in his cancer research.

Despite his earlier notice by the U.S. military, the recognition of his contribution in the area of treating radiation-induced illnesses has largely waned. After the Chernobyl nuclear plant meltdown, Revici unsuccessfully offered his services in a letter to a Soviet emissary of the USSR. Not surprisingly, his offer fell on deaf ears. With much fanfare, genuinely caring physicians with higher public relations quotients volunteered their services to perform bone marrow transplants for Chernobyl victims.

In response, Revici pointed out, in a revision of a paper he had written years earlier, why the chosen approach of using bone marrow transplants to save Soviet radiation victims would not work. Revici noted that the project was doomed to failure because, "So long as [abnormal fatty acids] are in the body, they will act against transplanted bone marrow cells." Sure enough, bone marrow transplants have proven to be ineffective as a treatment against radiation poisoning.

To date more than ten thousand Russians have died as a result of the Chernobyl accident. Many of those affected have been young children due to the fact that radiation seems to take its greatest toll on the very young.

In his paper Dr. Revici provided a few examples of the effect of his treatment for radiation burns and sickness:

> Successful results in humans were seen in cases of proctitis, esophagitis and skin burns, which had not healed in months or even years, [all of which] responded well to the above agents. For example, 20 children with radiation skin burns following an accident in which the filter had been left off the x-ray machine were treated successfully.... [A] recent case of radiation induced esophagitis with a total incapacity to drink even water was enabled to eat meat following a 24-hour treatment.

On August 11, 1995 a Washington Post editorial took note that the average life span of the Russian people had declined markedly since 1987, an occurrence that is not even seen in third-world countries. The editorial commented that the sharp downturn was due to a combination of environmental causes and a lack of adequate available medical treatment. While the Chernobyl incident is only one of many contributors to the sharp drop in the average life span of the Russian population, the lives of many people—young and old—might have been saved if n-butanol had been made available to them.

It was not only the Soviet government that overlooked Revici's contributions. In 1950 Revici gave a formal lecture in London on his findings concerning the abnormal fatty acid structures he had discovered. Eleven years later he wrote extensively about those findings in his book.

Thirty-two years after Revici's lecture in London, Bengt Samuelsson won a Nobel Prize for his research on the same topic. To add further irony to the chronology of events, Samuelsson merely identified and described the process of abnormal fatty acids. Revici not only described it, he developed several successful treatments for the abnormality.

A. R. Salman, M.D., who has reviewed both scientists' work in this area, has stated that the two works are "one and the same." In comparing the two works, Dr. Salman found Revici's version to be the better of the two, "It is clearer and more detailed."

The impact of the Revici/Samuelsson discovery has recently begun to make an impression on the wider public with the release of the important bestseller, *The Zone*, by Dr. Barry Sears. In his book Sears repeatedly credits Samuelsson's prize-winning research as being the foundation for his own findings. For example:

> When the 1982 Nobel Prize in Medicine was awarded for eicosanoid research, it gave rise to a new and different perspective on disease.* Using this paradigm we can link many, if not all disease states in a new and unified picture....For some that could mean heart disease, for others cancer, arthritis or obesity.

---

* Eicosanoids are the class of hormones under which Samuelsson's research fell and for which he was awarded his Nobel Prize. In particular Samuelsson focused on leukotrienes, which are one of the "abnormally conjugated trienic fatty acids" Revici discovered.

In addition to genetic, anti-aging and hormonal factors, Dr. Sears also points out, "…[the] Zone-favorable diet is based on the 1982 nobel Prize in Medicine, which demonstrated the importance of eicosanoids in controlling how the human body functions." Through his book Sears has helped to substantiate one of the important pieces of the puzzle which Dr. Revici has put together.*

Another important application of structure to function is seen in Revici's use of compounds with special *twin formations*. Twin formations are electrical connections between atoms that share either a double-positive or a double-negative bond. While most connections between atoms occur between a negative and a positive bond, a twin formation occurs when two adjacent atoms within a molecule both have either a positive or a negative charge.

The energy potential of the twin formation is analogous to holding two magnets together that are fighting back. It requires an extra force to overcome the tendency of the magnets to push themselves away. In the case of atoms sharing these types of double positive or double negative bonds, an extra amount of energy exists.

As an example, Revici points to the ability of certain normal fatty acids to lock onto oxygen due to their twin-formation structure. In a normal fatty acid the structure generates an energy force between the two formations that helps the fatty acid to utilize the oxygen molecule.

One fatty alcohol, glycerol, has a triplet formation, which makes it especially effective in counteracting the problems caused by abnormal fatty acids, according to Revici. Revici has identified other triplet lipid formations as well.

A third way Revici's knowledge of physical chemistry has come into play has been in his selection of medicines. In many cases he found it useful to attach a single chemical element to a compound that could directly attack a tumor or other condition. For example, the element selenium is known to be an excellent anti-oxidant, which means it pre-

---

* While Sears focuses on the powers of essential fatty acids, his book provides less information on their antagonists—the sterold and fatty alcohols, which are the other half of Revici's dualistic approach to disease.

vents oxygen from being robbed prematurely from the system.

Selenium is considered to be extremely toxic, however. Its toxicity has presented real problems for nearly a hundred years. August von Wasserman, M.D., who is best known for developing the Wasserman test to detect syphilis, also used selenium to treat cancer in animals— with some promising results. Others who later followed him in that approach ran into difficulty when treating humans, however, due to the extreme toxic reactions experienced by the patients. Since then, selenium has fallen into general disfavor as a cancer treatment in the mainstream scientific community.

Overdoses of selenium cause dramatic and easily identifiable symptoms in humans and can even result in the death of the patient. As the most recent Surgeon General's Report on Health and Nutrition points out, "Selenium is one of the most toxic essential elements." Yet Revici has given patients doses of selenium thousands of times above the level considered safe without any signs of a toxic reaction.

How does he do it? The answer lies in the proper use of physical chemistry. Revici developed a method of chemically incorporating the selenium into the middle of oil-based lipidic compounds. By positioning the selenium in the middle of a lipidic molecule, the water-soluble element was placed in a cocoon of a non-water-soluble substance, thereby preventing toxicity as a result of the element prematurely disconnecting from the lipid prior to its destination.

To get a clearer picture of the difference between a selenium molecule on the end of a lipid molecule compared to one in the middle of a molecule, a far-fetched analogy might be in order. Most people keep their televisions inside their homes. For a thief to get to it, he would generally need to go through the door. If the television were located on the front porch, access by a thief would be much more easily accomplished. Just as the walls and doors act as a buffer to a would-be thief, lipids act as a buffer to the water molecules in the body. Meanwhile, the homeowner with the proper key easily unlocks the door. Similarly, the lipids are easily unlocked at the site of abnormally configured lipids.

How important is the positioning of the element inside the lipid molecule rather than at the end? One answer is to recall how the

"Dade County Man" became the "Dead County Man" in the example above. Small changes in position can be very important.

The combination of the right lipid with the proper element allows a one-two punch that can be extremely effective in treating cancer, AIDS and a number of other conditions. Revici has used the element-within-a-lipid technique with quite a few elements, some for treating alkaline imbalances and others for acid imbalances.

One particularly powerful use of the element-within-a-lipid medicine comes into play in the treatment of brain tumors. The brain has a protective device known as the blood-brain barrier. It keeps noxious substances from entering that vital organ. Lipids pass through the blood-brain barrier, however. Once the lipid finds its way to the tumor, it unlocks the incorporated element which can then attack the malignant cells. Revici has many long-term brain tumor survivors, some of whom you will read about later.

The precise and intricate configurations of Revici's medications came about, not from guess work, but from sound concepts applied by a knowledgeable scientist. For example, in Revici's study of lipids, he found the existing definitions of lipids to be unsatisfactory. In addition to redefining the term scientifically, he also worked on a precise mathematical definition of lipids. To accomplish that task, he enlisted the help of Dr. Jacques Mariani, a mathematician at the Institute for Advanced Studies at Princeton.

In one of the Princeton libraries reside copies of a series of letters between Mariani and Albert Einstein discussing the challenge of producing a mathematical definition for lipids, up to their final breakthrough.*

During that time Revici met with Einstein, and they discussed Revici's theory of Hierarchic Organization. Because Hierarchic

---

* The final mathematical equation, which has no less than five Greek symbols along with a variety of computational requirements, was to be discussed in a separate chapter in Revici's 1961 book. The only copy of the draft of the particular chapter was given to another mathematician to proofread. While it was in possession of the proofreader, a housekeeper discarded it. Revici never attempted to reconstruct the chapter. The equation survived, however, as an end note with one paragraph of discussion included.

Organization was one of the main topics of discussion, one could understand how Einstein might have been favorably impressed with Dr. Revici's mind.

Revici's ability to manipulate chemical structures has played an important part in his developing over 100 different medications. Some stop the craving for heroin and cocaine in three days. Others reverse the symptoms of AIDS. One allowed a catatonic schizophrenic, who hadn't spoken in years, to carry on a normal conversation within minutes. Another stops the desire for alcohol. Another drug stops arterial bleeding and prevents shock. Yet another helps people to quit smoking.

Many of these medications have existed for twenty, thirty, forty or even fifty years. None of them are generally available to the public in the U.S., except at Revici's office. To most of us, this can be difficult to understand. If Revici's medications are as effective as they are claimed to be here, why aren't they widely available? That question may start to loom larger when the reader sees in the next chapter the many advances Revici has made in the treatment of AIDS.

7

A Curative Approach: Revici's Success with AIDS

"Dr. Revici's research in lipids and their therapeutic application in HIV infection and AIDS has proved to be extremely effective — a fact reflected by improvement of 'T' lymphocyte counts and clinical conditions as well. His work is definitely promising and opens vast areas of investigation and study in the field."

CAROLINA STAMU, M.D.

In 1987, the *Townsend Letter for Doctors* published an article Dr. Revici had written two years earlier. In it he discussed the AIDS syndrome and his method of treatment for it.

Within the 5,000-word article, Revici touched on at least fifty-four discoveries he had made regarding or related to the functions of human and animal anatomy. Several of those medical discoveries have the potential to advance the method of treating AIDS significantly. Revici described AIDS as a condition with four major components — a quadruple pathology, as he called it. An infected individual might manifest only one or all four levels of the pathology. Each additional level of the disease complicates the chance of success in treating the condition.

In short, the disease begins with a virus which, if left unchecked, contributes to a generalized susceptibility to localized bacterial infections. Those localized infections will then proceed into secondary infections which are sometimes accompanied by certain types of malignancies. In its final stages a systemic condition characterized by an "intensive" lipidic imbalance ensues.

By using a quadruple approach, approximately 50% of his AIDS patients have shown objective improvement according to indicators such as the elevation of the Helper/Suppressor Ratio (H/S Ratio) or an increase in the T_4 cell count. In some of his patients the H/S Ratio returned to normal or near normal. In contrast, the record for increasing the H/S Ratio through conventional means is universally poor and is associated with an AIDS cure rate that presently approaches 0%.

Several case histories were included in the Townsend article, such as that of a 33-year-old male. Before treatment the patient suffered from a very poor T_4 cell count of 188, chronic fatigue and a 15-pound weight loss. Eleven months after the start of treatment his T_4 count had risen to about 950, an increase of over 500%. Meanwhile, his H/S Ratio jumped from .8 to 1.6, a 100% increase. His fatigue subsided, and he regained the weight he had lost.

According to Revici, the first of the four characteristics of AIDS occurs at the viral level. As the reader will recall, viruses correspond to the subnuclear compartment in Revici's system of Hierarchic Organization. As we have seen, viruses can be controlled by the administration of special fatty acids.

To prove his hypothesis regarding the role of fatty acids in the control of viruses, Revici injected a large number of rabbits with either fatty acid lipids or with sterol lipids given just under the skin. Twenty-four hours later, the "prepared skin" sites were exposed to a virus. Revici reported, "For the virus inoculation very clear results were obtained...." Revici wrote that the sterols, "exerted a promoting (enhancing) effect on viral replication," but the fatty acids, "showed a profound inhibitory effect, suggesting a role for these substances in anti-viral activity."

The experiment demonstrated that Revici's hypothesis regarding the relationship between viruses and bacteria was correct: the fatty acids exhibited a natural defense activity to control viruses. The sterols —which are the antagonists of fatty acids—promoted viral activity.

Armed with that knowledge, Revici began treating his AIDS patients with fatty acids for the purpose of stopping the activity of the AIDS virus. According to his report in the Townsend Letter, treatments with his fatty acid medications were effective and long lasting:

> After the other manifestations have been controlled *[an anti-viral treatment] was seen to keep patients entirely without symptoms for years. In addition, with such treatment, changes in the helper-suppressor ratio from abnormal to normal have been obtained,* together with the disappearance of most clinical signs of the disease. (emphasis added)

By the time Bob* came to see Dr. Revici in July of 1986, he had experienced three to four years of chronic diarrhea and was suffering from mild dementia, a not uncommon condition among AIDS patients. He weighed 155 pounds. Six months prior to seeing Revici, he had been diagnosed as positive for hepatitis B and was also found to be HIV positive. Bob continued to see Revici regularly for the next two years.

Seven years after his first visit with Revici, Bob was seen by a physician in the San Francisco area. By then Bob weighed 207 pounds. The doctor gave him a thorough exam, but found everything to be normal except for a possible hernia and a "minimal" enlargement of a lymph gland in his neck, according to a copy of the doctor's medical report.

The second part of the quadruple pathology that Revici describes occurs at the bacterial level. According to Revici's theory of Hierarchic Organization, bacteria correspond to the nuclear compartment.

Upon their initial visit to Revici, most patients with AIDS would also have signs of bacterial infections along with their viral symptoms. It appears that when the AIDS virus is left unchecked, it will induce an attack on the lipidic defense system at the bacterial level, thereby allowing the AIDS patient to be susceptible to a great variety of bacte-

---

* All patient names used in this chapter are pseudonyms.

rial infections.

Revici identified a class of lipids which he suspected to be anti-bacterial. Revici found that these lipids, known as phospholipids, when administered orally, would provide astounding protection to infant mice that were exposed to the tuberculin bacteria, anthrax or E-coli bacteria. The death rate for the *untreated* mice was 100% for both tuberculosis and anthrax. For the mice infected with E-coli, the death rate was 86%. In contrast, the mice *treated* with phospholipids had almost perfect protection. Of that group, only 8 to 12% of the mice infected with the tuberculin bacteria died. Furthermore, none of the mice exposed to either the anthrax or E-coli bacteria died after treatment with phospholipids.

According to Revici, the results obtained with the administration of phospholipids to AIDS patients were very good:

> Subjective changes were often seen *within an hour* after injection of these lipids. In pneumocystitis pneumonia *[a killing factor in AIDS] and other opportunistic infections, manifest favorable changes were often obtained in less than 24 hours.* (emphasis added).

Based upon his laboratory and clinical research Dr. Revici concluded that the loss of certain specific phospholipids, "represent the missing factor in the special pathogenesis of AIDS."

For example, Mike, age 34, began treatment for tuberculosis in December of 1982. The following summer it was determined that he had AIDS and a T_4 count of 575. A little more than two years later—with continued treatment—his T_4 count had nearly tripled to 1,552—a level considered to be completely normal. His H/S Ratio rose from .7 to 1.24, a 77% increase. The patient gained ten pounds while his symptoms of chronic fatigue and swollen lymph glands disappeared. During treatment, Mike's tubercular lesion also became smaller in size.

As we have seen in previous chapters, abnormal lipids can play a direct role in cancer formation as well as in primary viral infections. When the damage in the second compartment remains unchecked, an AIDS patient's condition will deteriorate into the third level of the quadruple pathology. Revici describes the third component as one being marked by secondary opportunistic infections and a tendency to develop lymph cancer and/or Kaposi's sarcoma, a deadly skin cancer.

To combat the effects of a disease that has reached this stage, patients are treated with a combination of lipidic medicines. Patients are given fatty acids for their viral infection, and one of the phospholipidic agents for their bacterial infections. For the third level of the disease, either anabolic or catabolic lipids incorporated with a chemical element are provided to combat the more generalized breakdown of the lipidic defense system. It is at this stage of the disease that the encapsulated elements such as potassium, copper, selenium, or zinc are needed to help stabilize the condition.

Although Revici says that AIDS is a "very difficult" disease to treat successfully, the following two cases demonstrate that he is sometimes able to help AIDS patients a great deal.

Jim, a 38-year-old male, was confirmed to have Kaposi sarcoma of the lip, based on a biopsy performed prior to his first appointment with Revici in December of 1983. He had also suffered from a "persistent diarrhea" during the previous eight months. Four months later a second tumor appeared on his right arm, but by April both lesions had disappeared and the patient "was feeling very well."

The patient discontinued treatment in November. Three weeks later another cancerous lesion appeared. A lipid containing selenium was prescribed "with rapid resolution of the lesion." By October of 1985, Jim's T_4 count had climbed 194 points, an increase of 52%. His H/S Ratio was up 62%. By the time Revici's article went to press, Jim was continuing his treatment with anti-bacterial lipids being added to his protocol.

Ted first saw Revici in December of 1983 with a low grade fever, and swollen lymph glands under his armpit and in his neck. Diagnosed with AIDS, Ted experienced chronic fatigue and a loss of 15 pounds. Ted's spleen was also enlarged. During treatment he experienced several bouts of "upper respiratory infections and bronchitis with chills and fever from which he recovered as the result of more intensive administration of the [anti-bacterial] lipids. During the course of treatment [Ted] gained 15 pounds..." His chronic fatigue went away while the swelling in his lymph nodes disappeared, as did the swelling of his spleen. "He has felt completely well since the Spring of 1985, without recurrence of symptoms," Revici would write in the Townsend article.

The fourth level of pathology is seen only in the sickest AIDS patients as a result of the illness progressing beyond the first three levels. In this phase the patient manifests an extreme systemic lipid imbalance. Although the prognosis for these patients is guarded, the quality of their lives can often be dramatically improved. In some cases, phenomenal recoveries have been reported.

For example, Marcus Cohen, director of the Coalition To Increase Medical Empowerment, told me the story of an AIDS patient who was expected to die within twenty-four hours. The patient "couldn't hold his [bladder], and he couldn't hold his feces." Revici gave the man an injection. The man made a stunning recovery. With continued treatment, "He lived two more years with a much improved quality of life."

By the mid 1980's Revici found that AIDS patients often had intracellular deficiencies of either copper or potassium. The copper deficiency was common in acid imbalances and potassium deficiencies were common in the alkaline imbalances. The intracellular deficiency was caused by abnormal lipid formations which would dump the unused potassium or copper into the blood. (In fact, a blood serum test might indicate an excessive level of the element.) Revici predicted that adding either a potassium or a copper compound would have little effect in correcting the deficiency because the abnormal lipid formations wouldn't be able to hold onto the needed element.

To correct the lipid imbalance while providing the needed missing element, Revici decided to take a two-fold approach by incorporating the needed element into the middle of a lipidic substance. The central location of these lipid-attached elements prevented them from separating from the compound prior to reaching the intracellular compartment where they would be needed. In this way, the intracellular lipidic imbalance would be corrected and the necessary element would then be available for use within the cell.

Revici has found in a number of AIDS cases that excess copper in the blood serum is caused by an inability of the cytoplasm to use the element properly due to a malfunction of an anabolic lipid in the intracellular compartment. To get at the source of the problem, the treatment involves administering a catabolic lipid containing the element of copper to correct the lipid imbalance at the cytoplasmic level which will then allow the copper to be used properly within the cell.

Similarly, Revici found that in AIDS patients an excess of potassium in the blood serum was usually due to a catabolic lipid malformation within the intracellular compartment which causes the potassium to be sloughed off into the extracellular compartment. In that situation an anabolic lipid containing the potassium element would be administered to correct the imbalance which would then allow the potassium to be properly utilized.

In August of 1994, the New York Times and the Washington Post both reported the news that a team of University of Georgia scientists headed by Professor Will Taylor had demonstrated that the trace mineral selenium has a role in delaying the onset of AIDS. According to the research, the AIDS virus is contained within the person's cell as long as any selenium remains in the cell. Once the selenium is depleted, however, the virus "breaks out" spreading to the rest of the body, looking for more selenium and, in a sense, sucking the life out of its victim in the process.

The Taylor study is considered to be a significant breakthrough in the long march to find a satisfactory cure for AIDS. The New York Times article quoted Professor Gerhard Schrauzer: "It's very exciting work. It shows we must look at all aspects of the virus, and treatments that include simple nutritional agents."

Taylor's findings also help to confirm Dr. Revici's use of selenium for AIDS patients since 1978. Revici has also found that his lipid-based selenium compounds are useful for treating anabolic pattern symptoms, especially lymphomas and Kaposi's sarcoma, in AIDS patients.

In a wide-ranging telephone interview with the author, Professor Taylor also noted that the deadly Ebola virus has eight receptors to attack intracellular selenium, whereas the AIDS virus has only one. He pointed to the larger number of selenium receptors of the Ebola as a possible explanation for the rapidity of death caused by that virus.

Taylor went on to say that a rarer but even more deadly African virus has 16 selenium receptors, which might provide a clue to its virulence as well.

The challenge Taylor and others face is how to provide enough selenium to keep these deadly viruses contained within the cell without poisoning the patient. Fortunately, Revici's selenium compounds do not become toxic because of the selenium's position in the middle of the compound. That positional feature means that Revici's lipidic selenium compounds might be the drug of choice to treat the virulent types of viruses noted by Taylor.

The importance of solving the threat of viral and bacterial epidemics is explored at length by Laurie Garrett in her critically acclaimed book, *The Coming Plague*. The Pulitzer-Prize-winning writer makes a compelling argument that the populations of the world are particularly vulnerable to an epidemic from any number of viral and bacterial sources at the present time.

In the search for anti-viral drugs, modern medicine has recognized that there are too many kinds of viruses, and that they mutate too quickly to warrant much of an attempt to try to develop anti-viral agents. The huge variety of viruses makes the challenge of developing specific anti-viral medicines a virtual impossibility. Still, the scientific community has reported a number of deadly viral outbreaks in recent years. They are also learning about new strains of what may be a more dangerous form of the AIDS virus.

The closest modern medicine has come to stopping viruses is to develop vaccines. Vaccines work by injecting a dead virus into the patient, which allows the patient to develop an immunity to that particular strain of virus. Vaccines offer little or no protection against mutated strains of the injected virus, however. Furthermore, other than Revici's medications, there is presently no cure for individuals who have already contracted a virus.

It would appear that modern medicine is ill prepared for a massive viral outbreak like the ones that Taylor and Garrett caution us about, or from other as yet undiscovered viral strains. If the likelihood of catastrophic outbreaks made by Garrett and others is correct, it would seem imperative that Revici's anti-viral medications become a priority for the nation and the world.

Although one of the miracles of modern medicine has been the development of antibacterials, we have also seen a limit to their effectiveness. More and more physicians are uncovering bacterial infections that are resistant to conventional anti-bacterial medicines.

Billions of years of evolution and Revici's research demonstrate that fatty acids are impervious to the threats of a virus. It is unlikely, therefore, that viruses would be able to develop a resistance to Revici's fatty acids any time soon. The same reasoning tells us that phospholipids should also remain effective against bacterial infections.

Should an epidemic strike, it will be crucial to have at our disposal medicines that are not subject to loss of effectiveness due to mutations. Even more importantly, it will be critical to have anti-viral and anti-bacterial medicines that can be effective against a broad spectrum of viruses and bacteria. Revici's compounds meet those challenges.

Although much of Revici's work in the anti-viral area has been with AIDS patients, the basis for that work is more basic and strikes at the fundamental nature of viruses, bacteria and malignancies. So far, the application of his theory of Hierarchic Organization regarding AIDS has often proved beneficial, according to Dr. A. R. Salman:

> When I worked with Revici in the early and mid-eighties, I saw terminal AIDS patients who improved. Some lived almost normal lives. Recently, I talked to a former Revici patient who had AIDS more than ten years ago. Back then he had diarrhea and pneumocystitis. Now he's fine.

As Dr. Revici has said regarding his own discoveries, "What I discovered, I *recognized*. It may take others five, ten or twenty-years. I didn't make it up. It is a fact."

As yet, Revici's discoveries in these two important areas of viruses and bacteria await rediscovery by the rest of the scientific community. Whether or not we and the world community will have the luxury of the twenty years offered by Dr. Revici, remains to be seen.

8

You Don't Have to Bleed to Death and Other Good News

---

*"Vomiting, nausea, belching and retching ceased
almost at once, and there was no further evidence
of bleeding for the next 36 hours."*

EMANUEL REVICI, M.D. AND ROBERT RAVICH, M.D.
ANGIOLOGY, DECEMBER 1953

Anyone unfortunate enough to have a serious accident while driving
down the autobahn in Germany has a line of defense we don't have in
the United States.

Two of the major causes of death in car accidents are blood loss and
shock. An artery gets nicked or severed, and the heart pumps the blood
out through the breech. Sometimes the bleeding is visible—sometimes
it's internal. Oftentimes victims will go into shock as a result of their
blood loss. Both blood loss and shock can—and frequently do—kill.

The difficulty with effectively treating shock due to bleeding comes
from two countervailing, life-threatening conditions that occur at the

same time. The first is loss of blood. The second is a drop in blood pressure. If the blood pressure is increased, it can increase blood loss—causing death. Yet if blood pressure drops, both brain damage and/or death can result. Unless the damaged artery can be located and the blood flow stanched, no single treatment available in the U.S. effectively deals with the simultaneous effects of blood loss and falling blood pressure.

With more than 40,000 people dying each year from auto accidents in the U.S. alone, loss of blood and shock are serious challenges that emergency teams face every day.

There are several other ways that people can experience serious blood loss. For example, malignant tumors will suddenly cause profuse bleeding when an invasive cancer eats through an arterial blood vessel or when the tumor itself ulcerates. Such an event is frequently life threatening. Modern medicine is only partially successful in dealing with these conditions, and loses more times than it wins.

Another potentially serious condition is known as *seventh-day bleeding*. After having plastic surgery of the nose, patients will sometimes develop sudden bleeding from their nasal passages. Although the incidence of seventh-day bleeding has been greatly reduced with the administration of antibiotics, according to Revici, its prevention is still a potential problem for plastic surgeons and their patients. In a small percentage of cases the bleeding can become life threatening.

Certain kinds of heart surgery are sometimes associated with a condition called seventh-day chest pain, which Revici has found to be caused by cardiac infarction (heart attack). The *Mosby Medical Encyclopedia* describes an *infarct* as "a localized area of decay in a tissue.... An infarct can resemble a red swollen bruise, because of bleeding and an accumulation of blood." Modern medicine also treats this potential condition with antibiotics which prevents many, but not all, incidents. Some patients die from this condition. With the large number of heart surgeries performed, seventh-day chest pain and its complications are important concerns among physicians.

An effective treatment for all of the above conditions was developed by Dr. Revici in the mid 1940's as the result of his research. The same medicine that proved useful in the treatment of radiation-induced ill-nesses proved useful for bleeding and shock as well. The wary reader might wonder about an elixir that supposedly has so many different uses. Revici attempted to answer that question early in his book:

"Upon close analysis, nature, which appears to be so greatly var-ied, turns out, in fact, to be based on only a few very fundamental constituents, and it is the manner in which these constituents are bound together...which provides variety.

"And it would not appear too much to expect that, if nature's seemingly infinite variety stems from the organization of only a few constituents, then organization itself might also be achieved through a few, relatively simple fundamental patterns. If so, *such patterns...could be of primary importance to [a] better understanding of a host of problems."* (emphasis added).

Besides theorizing why different biological functions might have similar etiologies, Revici also performed yeoman research in the lab to establish the connections. Still, the best proof is, "How did the patient respond?" So we'll take a look at that also.

N-butanol stops arterial blood loss without clotting while maintain-ing the person's normal blood pressure. In the case of arterial bleeding, the contraction of the artery takes effect only at the site of injury. It has no effect on uninjured arteries.

In Germany the drug is available at most pharmacies and is called "Hemostipticum Revici." For many years every Mercedes-Benz sold in Germany came with a package of Hemostypticum Revici in its first-aid kit. It is also carried by the rescue squads in Germany. Hemostypticum contains an n-butanol solution with small amounts of organic acids.

The drug also prevents and reverses the condition of shock. As early as 1961, Revici described three categories of shock: *superacute shock, acute shock,* and *state-of-shock.*

According to Revici's research, superacute shock manifests itself in the central nervous system and occurs immediately, often resulting in death. Acute shock usually develops within thirty minutes from the time of a traumatic event and can also cause death if not treated immediately. State-of-shock takes much longer for its onset, often not showing its effects until approximately seven days after a traumatic event, yet it can cause a heart attack. Because of its delayed onset, state-of-shock often goes unrecognized as the cause of the patient's condition.

Of course there is a difference between a condition being recognized and its existence as a phenomenon. Everyone knows of someone who has suffered a heart attack a week after experiencing a traumatic event. Revici's research established laboratory evidence of this phenomenon of state-of-shock.

In animal studies conducted by Revici, superacute shock attacked the nerve cells, while acute shock attacked the tissues. State-of-shock attacks the organs and systems. Among other findings Revici found that all categories of shock caused a darkening of the blood due to damage to the red blood cells caused by an influx of fatty acids.

In the animal studies, he found a common event in all three types of shock. Just like in the radiation studies, all three types of shock produced high levels of abnormal fatty acids and a correspondingly high oxalic acid index. In further studies n-butanol proved to be an effective treatment for all three types of shock. It also prevented the occurrence of acute shock and state-of-shock when administered before their onset.

N-butanol can also play a role in the treatment of cancer patients. In 1950, the American Cancer Society sent Revici's chief associate, Robert Ravich, M.D., an acceptance letter to publish in their magazine, *Cancer*, a study of the effects of n-butanol in stopping spontaneous arterial bleeding in advanced cancer patients. The article detailed some astonishing results. The ACS never published the article, however. Finally, in December of 1953 the less widely read publication, *Angiology*, did publish the article. The famed heart surgeon, Michael E. de Bakey, M.D., was one of the editors of *Angiology* at the time.

The study was comprised of 600 cancer patients, 7% of whom developed severe bleeding problems as a result of their cancer. In the group of 18 bleeders who did not receive treatment with n-butanol, 12 bled to death. In the group treated with n-butanol, only 1 out of 25 patients who had experienced arterial bleeding died from it.

N-butanol would typically stop the bleeding for one or more days, but wasn't a permanent cure for the bleeding episodes in cancer patients. As a result some of the cancer patients treated with n-butanol had numerous occurrences of sudden bleeding during the course of their illness. In that group of 25 patients, episodes of arterial bleeding occurred on "more than 300 occasions." Despite the numerous recurrences of arterial bleeding, however, the n-butanol treatment was effective in saving the patients' lives on all but one occasion.

The Revici/Ravich article provided ten case histories which were described as being typical of the n-butanol cases. One case from the study, regarding a fifty-two-year-old female, is illustrative:

> She suddenly began to vomit copious amounts of coffee-ground material followed by large amounts of blood followed [by] clots.... Five cc of n-butanol in saline solution was injected intravenously. Vomiting, nausea, belching and retching ceased almost at once, and there was no further evidence of bleeding for the next 36 hours. On several occasions thereafter, vomiting of coffee-ground material recurred and was controlled with 5-10 cc of n-butanol solution...

The effectiveness of n-butanol in seventh-day-post-operative nasal bleeding was demonstrated in a major study by Dr. S. Sher, a plastic surgeon. The study included nearly 2,000 nasal surgeries where antibiotics were not used. Seventh-day bleeding is seen in up to 10% of post-operative nasal surgeries unless antibiotics are administered as a preventative.

Not one of the 2,000 patients developed severe bleeding when treated with n-butanol preventively. According to an end note in Revici's book, "In several cases where patients failed to follow instructions and did not continue taking butanol, hemorrhage resulted. In two cases [where] bleeding was relatively severe, the hemorrhage was brought under control by the intravenous injection of 10 to 20 cc. of the butanol solution."

Another condition that can be treated preventively with antibiotics is seventh-day bleeding following heart surgery. Revici says that seventh-day bleeding after either nasal or heart surgery is caused by an allergic reaction. Seventh-day chest pain after heart surgery and the associated death that sometimes occurs can also be prevented by treatment with n-butanol, according to Revici. One advantage of n-butanol over antibiotics is that most physicians would prefer to avoid their overuse. Another advantage is that n-butanol has no apparent side effects, whereas antibiotics do.

Not all tragedies are accidental or even physical. The illness of schizophrenia usually strikes its victims in their late teens and early twenties. Victims live with their disease until they die. No treatment has yet been found that comes even close to bringing them back to a normal life. Many of these lost souls split their time among mental institutions, the lock-up wards of hospitals, half-way houses, and the streets. When on the streets their tortured lives sometimes include lunching on half-eaten burger buns and chewy french fries. Their cycle of street-roaming freedom is often temporarily interrupted by forced hospitalization due to their recurring unlawful behavior. On occasion some schizophrenics, particularly males, can become quite violent.

One of the most fascinating potential uses of n-butanol may well be to treat schizophrenia. In the late 1940's Revici spent several mornings a week working with H. A. LaBurt, M.D., director of Creedmoor State Hospital, which is located in Queens, New York.

Over a period of three years, Revici tested over 27,000 urine samples from 27 patients with "advanced schizophrenia." Other tests were also conducted. According to Revici's book, "more than 135,000 tests were performed." From those studies urinary peroxides were found in 87% of the urine samples tested. Revici noted, "This appears to be highly significant when compared with only 2% positive values in subjects considered normal, and 4% in cancerous cases submitted to various treatments." From that work the urinary peroxide test was termed the "Revici Reaction" and could well be the first scientific demonstration of a biochemical connection in the disease of schizophrenia.

The schizophrenic patients were also found to suffer from an intense localized catabolic imbalance which produced a generalized anabolic reaction. The 27 patients were given very high doses of n-butanol by injection. The amounts prescribed for the study were two to five times the amounts given to cancer patients. An abstract of the results was published by Creedmoor Hospital in the "Creedmoor Annual Report" of 1949. According to the report:

> "The effect was immediately clear. Cases with complete mutism of long duration responded verbally to questions.... In some cases the satisfactory response continued for several days and in one case, for more than a week.

> "Research in schizophrenia has indicated the existence of a [lipidic imbalance] in all cases. Administration of lipobases has produced some improvement, while lipoacids have aggravated the symptoms."

Years later, Revici would testify in an administrative court about one of the schizophrenic patients who hadn't spoken in years. According to Revici, after receiving a single injection, the patient began to carry on a normal conversation and joked with the nursing staff.

The study was discontinued, however, because the extremely large doses produced inflammation of the vein on a few occasions. Transitory sleepiness was also noted in a few of the patients. No attempt was made to conduct a new study using smaller dosages. The failure to follow-up might be another dramatic example of Revici's lack of long-term interest in research not related to cancer. Even so, Revici's work was probably the first to demonstrate the existence of a physical imbalance in schizophrenia.

When I asked Dr. Revici about the 1940's experiment, he suggested that a lower dose given over the period of a month might produce similar positive results without the side effects.

The use of n-butanol and other lipobases to treat schizophrenics is a rich area for further research.

9

Magic Bullets for Drug Addiction and Alcoholism

"The results and what we witnessed [were] so unbelievable that the doctor from Municipal Hospital has now gone back on a daily basis in order to continue with this chance to see the miraculous results that have taken place."

REPRESENTATIVE CHARLES RANGEL, U.S. CONGRESSIONAL
SELECT COMMITTEE ON CRIME HEARING, APRIL 1971

There are two stories as to how Revici developed his treatment for drug addiction. Both accounts may have part of the truth in them. In the first story, told by Marcus Cohen, Revici noticed that his cancer patients could discontinue their use of narcotic drugs without experiencing withdrawal symptoms after they started on Revici's cancer medications. From that awareness Revici wondered if his medicines could also be used to break the addiction pattern in drug addicts.

There are two weaknesses in that account, however. Revici has known since the late 1930's that his medications usually eliminated the need for narcotics. Yet he didn't focus on implementing his drug addiction treatment until 1970. In fairness to Cohen's account, it is possible that Revici didn't show any interest in the drug addiction question due to his consuming interest in cancer research.

Another unanswered question from Cohen's explanation is, if that were so, why didn't Revici simply use his cancer drugs to treat drug addicts? Revici's method often allows the use of the same medicine for different diseases. Yet he developed a new compound specifically to treat drug addiction.

The late Daniel H. Casriel, M.D., a psychiatrist who founded the Daytop program for drug addicts, provided the second part of the story. Speaking before a U.S. Congressional committee concerned with the drug problem in the U.S., he testified about the way Revici came up with his formula, "He designed the drug with a piece of paper and a pencil."

Revici's own recollection of his invention, told in broken English, succinctly describes not only his approach to that particular matter, but also describes his approach to many of the scientific challenges that have faced him over the years. When he spoke, I was struck by the paradox between the softness of his voice and the power behind his few words. At the age of 98 Dr. Revici was not as loquacious as his earlier years. Yet the impact of his remarks seems to be undiminished either by his grammar or the small number of his words.

"At the time I realized the drug [problem] was very big," he said. "Maybe not so much today. But then, very big. That made me very interested, to help." As he has done with other biochemical puzzles, he would ponder the problem until he came upon the answer. "First, not so difficult, but then more difficult. And then—the solution!"

In April of 1971 Dr. Casriel explained in his testimony to the Congressional panel the various parts of the chain reaction that Revici determined to be an answer to the problem. Casriel told the panel that the body tends to overreact to an alkaloid drug, such as heroin or cocaine, by producing too much of a steroidal defense reaction.

Casriel then told the panel that the excess steroids produced in reaction to heroin latch onto the body, thereby robbing it of oxygen. The oxygen deficit causes pain in the user, "...similar to the type of pain and feelings you would get if a tourniquet were tied around your hand," he said. Casriel testified that when the addict is deprived of his drug, the localized acidosis also produces a generalized reaction, causing, "...[the] so-called cold turkey phenomena."

The development of a medication for addiction might have been easier for Revici than for other conditions because he knew that drug addiction caused an extremely alkaline reaction in the user's body. (Specifically, in a localized acidosis, the body sets up a generalized alkaline reaction.) As we have seen from Dr. Mann's remarks in Chapter 1, Revici's knowledge at the time regarding steroids was probably unmatched by anyone in the world. That advanced understanding, combined with his mastery of physical chemistry, enabled him to design a medicine that would stop the oxygen-robbing action of the illicit drug.

After formulating the new drug called "Perse" Revici tested it in his lab for efficacy and safety on "several thousands of laboratory animals," according to Casriel's testimony. Only then did he treat, "several thousand patients that he detoxified from heroin without any harmful effects."

Casriel added his own experience of administering Perse to his own drug addicted patients: "I have detoxified about 100 [patients] without any harmful effects whatsoever."

The Congressional committee learned from Dr. Casriel about the typical response of first-time Perse users, "[V]ery frequently the addict will say, 'My God! What did you give me? I feel like I got a fix, my stomach feels warm and good, my head feels clear, my head feels clear!'"

Casriel's testimony corresponds to what was reported the following year by David A. Loehwing in *Barron's* magazine regarding Perse:

> All the patients are drug addicts — heavy, long-term users....
> Normally, they should be climbing the walls, vomiting incessantly, clutching their bellies in the agony of withdrawal. Despite the assurances they have received, they seem surprised that they aren't suffering. "I feel fine, doctor", they all say, as Dr. Revici questions them. "No problems."

Casriel also related a personal experience he had with Revici's Perse. Casriel told the panel that he was particularly sensitive to alcohol,

"Normally two ounces of alcohol... will give me a drunk, and I fall asleep. I took two capsules of Perse and proceeded to drink eight ounces of scotch without any side effects of [slurred speech] or intoxication.... I was not drunk."

Casriel was not the only person impressed by the results of Perse on drug addicts. Congressman Charles Rangel, whose district includes areas of Harlem seriously impacted by drug addiction, was another. A streetwise politician, Representative Rangel had strong reservations when he first heard of the treatment method, "I felt the need to bring with me the administrator of the Harlem hospital drug rehabilitation program. That's how cynical I was."

Rangel was amazed by what he saw and told his fellow committee members:

> The results and what we witnessed [were] so unbelievable that the doctor from Municipal Hospital has now gone back on a daily basis in order to continue with this chance to see the miraculous results that have taken place.

Rangel was impressed enough to return more than once to Trafalgar Hospital. "I personally have gone back on several occasions to the clinic," he remarked at the hearing.

Revici was unable to attend the Congressional hearing due to his own illness. Rangel said that he wanted the panel to have a chance to get to know Revici, "[I hope] you will have the opportunity to really meet this very decent human being who I believe has made an outstanding contribution in this area."

In all, about three thousand heroin and methadone addicts were treated by Revici as well as about two hundred alcoholics. He developed a second drug called "Bionar"—a combining of the words "biology" and "narcotics,"—which worked equally well.

Perse contains the element selenium which is still considered by the FDA and NIH to be a highly toxic trace element. However, Revici had typically *injected* doses of selenium that were several thousand times the dose considered safe by mouth, without any side effects. His advanced knowledge of physical chemistry enabled him to produce a safe compound from a substance previously believed to be toxic.

Revici's research had demonstrated that there were four types of selenium compounds. Some forms were extremely toxic, but the form he used was nontoxic at the levels he used in his treatments. Professor Gerhard Schrauzer concurs with Revici's opinion on this matter, according to his court testimony on Revici's behalf.

Nonetheless, Revici developed Bionar, which is a selenium-free product, to make it easier to obtain FDA approval for the drug. (It might be noted that in the state of New York, physicians are allowed to use any substance they believe to be safe when treating patients. FDA regulations prevent unapproved medicines from being sent across state lines, however.)

For a medicine to be effective in the treatment of drug addiction, it should have several characteristics. First, it must work extremely quickly. "[W]ith addiction if you don't get some results in an hour or so, the patient becomes panicky," Dr. Revici told Barron's reporter, Loehwing. According to Dr. Casriel, Perse, "takes [effect in] about seven to fifteen minutes."

Second, the drug should be non-addictive. Replacing one addiction with another hardly does the patient much good. Methadone, for example, is an alkaloid that simply overpowers "the body's ability to produce more steroids," according to Casriel's testimony. For methadone addicts, Revici would sometimes add a butanol derivative to help clear out the effects of the methadone. From Revici's research it is clear that methadone creates a highly alkaline imbalance. Whether or not that sharply alkaline state could contribute to a host of lipidic defense illnesses, including cancer, arthritis and depression, ought to be examined.

Third, the medicine should be nontoxic. Perse and Bionar fit that requirement when given in the prescribed dosages. No side-effects were noticed with these remedies except that a few patients out of the thousands treated experienced a slight rash. Reducing the dosage eliminated that problem for those patients. This record is truly remarkable when one considers the average state of health of most drug addicts.

Fourth, the medication should not have to be taken for a long time.

Perse and Bionar usually detoxify heroin addicts in three days and methadone addicts in seven. The treatment for methadone addicts takes longer because it takes seven days to clear out the steroidal effects of the methadone addiction.

Fifth, the patient should lose his desire for the illicit drug. The patients universally reported that their desire for drugs disappeared after treatment with Perse or Bionar.

The only weakness of Perse and Bionar is that they don't remove the individual, familial and societal links to drug abuse. They do make the user much more receptive to corrective behavior, however, once the physical symptoms of addiction have disappeared. In other words, it is difficult to talk about the merits of a drug-free life when the patient's body is manufacturing excess steroids whose needs cry out to be met. On the other hand, a person whose drug-induced steroid production has been brought under control might be more than happy to take the next step to a better life.

Revici's remedies remove all the physical symptoms and cravings of drug addiction. They work quickly, cause no significant side effects, and are non-addictive.

DuPont Pharma recently received FDA approval for the treatment of alcohol addiction with the drug "naltrexone". DuPont originally introduced the drug they call ReVia for the treatment of heroin addiction. (The first four letters of ReVia, the same as the first four letters of Revici's last name, is not connected in any way to Revici.) ReVia fails to match up to either Perse or Bionar in several ways in the treatment of drug addiction.

ReVia must be taken for an extended period. It has caused side effects in a number of people. Long-term side effects of ReVia remain unknown for now and may be difficult to identify.

Care must be taken that it is used properly because, as the ReVia insert states, "ReVia is of proven value only when given as part of a comprehensive plan of management that includes some measure to ensure the patient takes the medication." That caution could be a major concern considering the long term usage required. Abrupt stoppage of the medication can be harmful or dangerous to the patient.

ReVia costs about four dollars a dose, whereas Perse cost about two cents per dose in 1971. With mark-up and distribution costs it still would not top a dollar even today. Furthermore, ReVia's true cost is four dollars a day for an extended period, perhaps for the rest of the patient's life.

ReVia is not recommended for patients with hepatitis or other liver ailments, yet drug addicts and alcoholics sometimes suffer from those conditions either clinically or subclinically. Nor is it recommended for people "currently dependent" on heroin or those "patients in acute [heroin] withdrawal," according to the ReVia package insert. Those restrictions on ReVia make it almost useless in transforming the average heroin addict into a drug-free person. The package insert warns that patients using ReVia who also take heroin risk the chance of coma or death. In contrast, a patient who relapses onto heroin during or after treatment with Revici's medicines is in no such danger. ReVia has no effect on the desire for cocaine.

Thus, twenty-five years after the invention of Perse and Bionar, the pharmaceutical companies have yet to find a medicinal heroin/alcohol treatment comparable to Revici's.

Perhaps the most important advantage of Revici's drug remedies was predicted by Casriel. He told the Congressional committee that the inherent limitations of methadone treatment would lead to an increase in cocaine addiction. The historical record of the past 25 years indicates that he was correct in his assessment.

Because ReVia cannot be prescribed for current users of heroin, methadone still remains the only accepted drug treatment remedy for *active* addicts because neither Perse nor Bionar were ever approved by the FDA. In Part IV, the reader will find out what may have prevented Revici's medicines from receiving FDA approval.

Meanwhile, as Dr. Casriel predicted, methadone has done little to resolve the drug crisis, as cocaine has replaced heroin on many street corners. The effects of crack cocaine have contributed heavily to a long list of societal problems. Ironically, the federal Drug Enforcement Agency has recently warned that heroin addiction is making a comeback.

10

From Heart Disease to Herpes: A Few Conditions That Respond to Lipid Therapy

So far, we have seen that cancer, AIDS, drug addiction, alcoholism, shock, PMS, schizophrenia, pathologically caused itching, and viral and bacterial infections might be amenable to lipidic therapy. Organized medicine is often reluctant to accept the possibility that a single substance or method can have an effect on seemingly unrelated conditions. It would be unfair to criticize Revici's method on that basis for a number of reasons.

His method differentiates one condition from another by using a number of different criteria. By using several different diagnostic lab tests, some of which Revici devised himself, he has been able to isolate at which hierarchic level a patient's condition is occurring. He can also pinpoint whether the condition is catabolic or anabolic, and can monitor that condition closely in the event that it switches to its opposite.

In addition, Revici doesn't use just one or two or even a few medications to treat his patients. In fact, he has over 100 patents for different medications he has developed.

Also, the notion held by organized medicine that each type of disease must have a separate cause, might not always be the best premise. For example, it is generally agreed that the condition of being significantly overweight is associated with and is a possible cause of a number of different health problems, including gall bladder disease, diabetes and heart trouble. Dr. Revici looks upon the lipid system as a separate defense *system*. Just as the immune system protects a person from any number of viruses and bacteria, the lipidic defense system can protect us from quite a few potentially harmful conditions as well.

If the physician's goal is to repair the total *system* rather than to attack each of the many illnesses that result from the impaired condition, fewer medications are likely to be required. Revici's method reinforces the basic building blocks of life, so it is not surprising that his method has application in the treatment of a myriad of diseases.

Using the house analogy once again, a house without a roof is open to numerous assaults from above: rain, hail, snow, sleet, falling tree limbs, squirrels, birds etc. One defense strategy would be to angrily occupy the top floor with an umbrella and a rifle to keep away some of the invaders, acting as though it were the squirrel's fault that we didn't have a roof. Another strategy would be to put a new roof in place—a single "medicine" for a myriad of undesirable situations.

The lipidic systems of the body act as a safety shield by keeping the noxious aspects of each level under control. In the lipidic defense system each compartment acts as the primary guardian against the noxious influences from the level below it.

If lipids play a role in a variety of functions at every level of human biological organization above the sub-nuclear, then it is also quite likely that they could be instrumental in correcting a large number of conditions. Indeed, Revici has been able to treat a number of seemingly unrelated conditions through the implementation of his guiding principles.

In 1983, at the age of eighty-seven, Revici prepared a twenty-two page summary of his "Research and Activity" which provides a snapshot of some of the diseases for which he has found a possible role for lipidic treatment. In the report, he briefly mentions a number of physical conditions that he has found to be connected to lipidic imbalances.

For example, he found that gastric ulcers, duodenal ulcers, ileitis and colitis are all strong acid-pain-pattern conditions.

According to Revici's clinical experience, cardiac insufficiencies are the result of a general catabolic imbalance, while irregular heart beats are caused by a localized anabolic imbalance. Herpes recurrences correspond to an anabolic imbalance while allergies and asthma have responded well to catabolic agents.

For example, in his book, Dr. Revici reported the case of Alexander Landis.* Revici states Mr. Landis, "had frequent attacks of asthma" for nearly five years, "which left him unable to work for the past year." Once treatment started, Mr. Landis was free of any asthma attacks for four months when he stopped taking the medication. Two weeks later, he had an asthma attack, followed by another attack the next day. "By resuming the medication, he has been free of symptoms for more than a year."

Migraines were found to be a catabolic condition of the membrane covering the brain and spinal chord. Bernard Welt, M.D., an ear, nose and throat specialist, conducted a study that included migraine patients. Dr. Welt treated a dozen migraine patients using Revici's method and medications, and the results were published in *Otolaryngology*, a peer-reviewed journal for ear, nose and throat physicians.

Every case of migraine was relieved by these treatments. Subsequent recurrences were also relieved by the medication. In the same study, 84% of vascular headaches resulting from a lipidic imbalance were relieved, and 75% of neuralgic headaches accompanied by a lipidic imbalance were also relieved.

As long ago as the 1930's, Revici's research demonstrated that osteoarthritis is an anabolic condition, while rheumatoid arthritis nor-

---

* All patient names used in this chapter are pseudonyms.

mally responded to treatment for catabolic disorders. Revici found that in cases of arthritis of either type, treatment based on the results of urinary surface tension provided the best effect even in the "most resistant cases." In regards to his treatment for arthritis, Revici wrote in his book:

> The simplicity of treatment, the total lack of undesirable side effects, and the long period of improvement after even brief treatment in some cases, indicates that this method is worthy of further investigation.

The case history of Nick Kramer is worth reviewing. Mr. Kramer's rheumatoid arthritis was so severe that he had been bedridden for six months prior to coming under Revici's care:

> The patient was entirely incapacitated, unable even to feed himself. Treatments with different cortisone preparations, ACTH, gold, etc., provided practically no relief of the severe pains.... [T]he patient made a dramatic recovery. Within a few days the patient was out of bed without pain and with full functional capacity of his arms and legs. While under treatment the patient went back to entirely normal activity.

According to Revici, high blood pressure is an anabolic condition and hardening of the arteries is a condition of the secondary part of the organ compartment—specifically the circulatory system—and responds to catabolic agents. Cholesterol buildup is indicative of anabolic excess in the cellular compartment.

Revici wrote in the 1983 summary that the lipidic forms of the element selenium "have given especially good results" for Alzheimer's Disease. It is also effective for memory deficiencies, according to Dwight McKee, M.D., a former associate of Dr. Revici.

Dr. Revici has had good success in treating both unipolar and bipolar depression with his lipidic treatments. He has also seen success in treating childhood retardation. According to Dr. McKee:

> His findings in retarded children indicated a lack of anabolic substances in the body. By administering the unsaponifiable fractions

of organs, especially brain, he obtained marked favorable, persisting changes in many such children.

"Sulfur compounds are very helpful in treating alcoholism and smoking," Revici also reported. He has used a specific medication he calls "ASAT" that he has found to be an excellent adjunctive treatment for cigarette addiction. It has proven to be quite helpful in a number of cases, according to Elena Avram, Revici's office manager for the past twenty-five years.

The always anabolic condition of convulsions has been treated effectively with lipidic sulfur and selenium compounds, according to Revici.

In addition to the already discussed n-butanol, certain sterols have been found to speed the healing of burns, cuts and wounds.

This is only a partial list of conditions that Dr. Revici has found to be treatable with lipidic medicines. It would be impossible to predict how many other conditions might also be determined to benefit from Revici's discoveries. Because of the fundamental nature of Revici's research, it is quite likely that researchers will find numerous other conditions that are also amenable to Dr. Revici's lipidic and Hierarchic Organization approaches.

Part II of this book has provided a look at only a portion of the findings by Dr. Emanuel Revici. For example, in his book Revici has written about the pharmacology of well over fifty elements and compounds by explaining the hierarchic level of organization for each one, their dualistic nature, their relationship to lipids, and their effect biochemically on patients and animals.

It appears that Dr. Cronk's prediction was conservative — Revici's leads could keep many scientists busy for a long time. In the next section you will meet some of the many patients who have not had to wait until Revici's work is rediscovered to benefit from it.

HIS PATIENTS

11

"That's Hokey"

*"After Dr. Smith saw how Issy's tumor
had shrunk, she ran down the hall and practically
knocked me down, she was so excited. She's a new doctor,
and she used to be supportive. But later she said,
'My license is on the line. I can't say anything.'"*

VERNON MORIN, ISSY'S FATHER, 1994

Issy's chemotherapy wasn't working. Three months before she saw Dr. Revici for the first time, Issy was treated at the Children's Hospital of Philadelphia (CHOP) with a potent medicine that, if used improperly, could burn skin. The drug was supposed to be flushed out of her system immediately after the treatment. But according to Issy's father, Vernon, that didn't happen for an hour-and-a-half. As a result her young body became a storage bin for the drug that her doctors had hoped would help cure her. Six hours after the episode, chunks of Issy's bladder came out with her bloody urine. But the cancer stayed.

One of her doctors at CHOP would later admit to Vernon that the drug had damaged Issy's bladder, her kidneys and her ureters, the little tubes that connect them. The damage to her kidneys meant that her body had a hard time keeping her salts in their proper balance. Without that balance she could go into shock and die.

It took a year before Vernon and Judy, Issy's mother, would find out about the extent of the damage—but not until after Issy went into shock and had to be rushed to an Atlantic City hospital. Even then the Morins were told of her dangerous salt imbalance only as the result of Vernon's own investigation into Issy's records.

All along, several of the doctors at CHOP had discouraged the Morins from taking Issy to see Dr. Revici for her neuroblastoma. When Vernon first brought up the topic of Revici's method to Issy's team of doctors, Dr. Audrey Evans, who is considered to be a top expert in neuroblastomas, told him, "That's hokey." Still, the doctors had nothing better to offer Issy at that point except pain killers to help ease the final weeks of her life. Little did those doctors know that Issy would recover to the point where she would spend many a summer's day playing and swimming in the river behind the family's small farm.

In fact, three weeks after the beginning of Revici's treatment, Issy's tumor had shrunk to half its original size. The young Dr. Kim Smith, one of the resident physicians at CHOP, became ecstatic when she saw the new pictures of the tumor. "She ran down the hall and practically knocked me down, she was so excited," reports Vernon. Months later she became more cautious, however. According to Vernon, "She said, 'My license is on the line. I can't say anything.'"

Vernon told this author that on more than one occasion the doctors from CHOP continually tried to convince him and his wife that Revici's method wasn't working, and that the tumor had returned. Despite their claims, an x-ray taken in February of 1994—after nine months of Revici's care—showed her tumor had shrunk to the size of a golf ball. The only remaining tumor-leg had become calcified, which prevented it from feeding on her body, squeezing her small intestine, or interfering with her spinal nerves.

Approximately one month later, Issy and her mother were involved in a serious auto accident. Judy received one broken and two bruised ribs. Issy's injury consisted of a seat belt bruise across her chest and abdomen just over the site of where her shrunken tumor lay.

Two months after the accident, Issy experienced renewed abdominal pain. Her condition gradually worsened to the point that Issy went into shock—after the Morins' ran into difficulty obtaining a physician-prescribed transfusion. She was rushed to the hospital in Atlantic City. According to Vernon, an attending physician wanted him to sign a "Do Not Resuscitate" consent form. Vernon told the doctor he would comply only if pictures were first taken to confirm that it was the tumor that was causing Issy's shock.

The physician resisted until Vernon informed the doctor that he would hold him personally responsible if his daughter died and an autopsy indicated some preventable cause of death. His hunch was correct. Although the pictures demanded by Vernon showed that Issy's tumor had sprouted a wispy three-inch finger, it certainly wasn't immediately life threatening.

It wasn't the cancer that had caused Issy's coma. Her unconscious condition had to be the result of something else. The doctors tried to convince the Morins the cancerous leg was ominous, nonetheless. When the pictures were later examined by a surgical oncologist at Dr. Revici's office, however, the Morins found out something a little different from what they had been told at the hospital. The new leg was only three inches long, not the six-foot rasping tentacle Issy's tumor had a year earlier. Because they can grow quickly, any new tentacle was not a good sign, but the new tumor growth wasn't what was causing her to go into shock.

Throughout the traumatic day and night of Issy's close brush with death, the doctors never volunteered the information regarding Issy's salt imbalance. In fact, Vernon discovered it as the result of his own detective work. He convinced a hospital worker to give him access to the computerized files of Issy's medical records. Only by studying them did Vernon discover the secret problem.

When confronted with the withheld information, one of the doctors reportedly told Vernon, "We didn't think you'd understand." It was at that time that the same doctor admitted there had been "chemo damage" done to Issy a year earlier which resulted in her inability to keep her salts balanced. According to Vernon the doctor told them, "She should have seen a nephrologist [a kidney specialist]."

The cancer drug that was used is so caustic that it comes with a warning to parents when changing their child's diapers. The warning includes instructions to parents to wear rubber gloves to protect their hands from getting burned by the chemical—the chemical that apparently hurt Issy's kidneys, bladder and urinary tract.

It was while she was at CHOP that Issy had previously told her parents she didn't want anymore treatments. She said she wanted to "be with the angels," according to her father.

While the debacle that occurred with the Morins is a dramatic example, it is all too typical of what the state of common treatment is today—and has been for most of this century. In too many cases neither the patient nor the family would have been told of the electrolyte imbalance. Yet, either the imbalance or the cancer would end up taking the patient to the grave. Make no mistake, if Issy's courageous parents hadn't demanded further proof and an explanation of their daughter's electrolytic imbalance, Issy could have died of shock that night far from home.

In contrast to the discouragement the Morins received from the medical personnel at CHOP, they found Revici's attitude to be more open and hopeful. When the Morins first took Issy to see Dr. Revici, they had also decided to try ayurvedic medicine, a holistic treatment popular in India. (The author Deepak Chopra, M.D., is one of the best known advocates of this system of medicine.) Vernon said that Revici welcomed the information and was quite curious about it.

Vernon says that when Issy went to visit Dr. Revici she liked to sit on his lap, but at CHOP, Issy would sometimes run away from the doctors screaming. After seeing Dr. Revici, Issy changed her mind about seeing the angels and said that she'd rather "stay here."

When Issy was at Children's Hospital, she had cancer in her abdomen, and she had it in her bloodstream. To a child her age, the tumor's size would be equivalent to an adult having a basketball-sized tumor riding on their adrenal gland. Few people could survive an ordeal like that.

You might say that Issy was a very lucky girl, because after seeing Dr. Revici, her cancer cells disappeared from her blood. The big tumor had lost its legs (until the car accident), and the former grapefruit-sized growth had shrunk to a fraction of its former size.

We know there are no guarantees in life, although we would all like to live a few more years. Most of us live a long life of sixty, seventy, eighty or even ninety years before we're done. But every so often among us are the ones who accomplish all they came here to do in just a few.

Issy bounced back for a while from the night of her shock. According to Vernon, the people at CHOP never did approve a nephrologist for Issy, and it became more and more difficult to keep her system working the way it had before. She died in her parent's bed in 1994 on an October afternoon cuddled by Judy and Vernon, sixteen months after the experts at CHOP told Issy's parents that Revici's method was hokey. Issy's last words, spoken moments before her death, were, "Mommy and Daddy, look at the beautiful birdies! Oh, they are so beautiful! No, I'm the birdie—I'm the birdie."

At his daughter's memorial service behind their home at the river where Issy liked to swim, Vernon saw a lone seagull land on one of the posts that held up the small dock from which Issy often jumped. Soon after, a flock of more seagulls passed over the river. The lone bird joined them and disappeared into the sky.

Later on, the reader will learn that the American Cancer Society and others say Revici's method is "unproven" and "without value." But then maybe they've never met a swimming, flying angel named Issy.

12

Robert Fishbein, M.D.:
Physician, Musician, Poet, and Patient

We took Mark to visit his newborn cousin in the hospital.
He was overwhelmed at all the infants and said,
"Dad, is this the infantry?"

I responded , "Well, in a way, I guess so..."

Mark said, "Where's the adultery?"

FROM *WHEN MARK WAS A WIDDLE BOY...*
AND *BEFORE MARK, THERE WAS LAUREN,*
COMPILED BY ROBERT E. FISHBEIN, M.D.

The above anecdote is but one of many coming from the mouths of Dr. Robert Fishbein's two children when they were young. Over the years Dr. Fishbein had recorded these sayings on three-by-five cards and has recently published them in a book. Three decades later the stories still bring back memories of the humorous yet thought-provoking perspectives of his children. The anecdotes are doubly priceless because he almost was not around to collect them.

The first indication of a problem came rather innocuously. He noticed a "slight twinge" in his head while walking down the hall of the hospital where he was working one Tuesday afternoon in late October of 1962.

He soon developed a stiff neck. He wondered fleetingly if he had meningitis. Flu-like symptoms gradually followed. By Friday he noticed that he was having difficulty driving his car, "My driving was drifting to one side." The next day his vision had become blurred, and he had developed a ferocious headache, "I banged my head against the tile wall in the bathroom. My daughter asked, 'Why is daddy crying so much?' "

Consultations with a couple of doctors during that week did little to stem the progress of what was originally thought to be a severe sinus infection. "On Sunday I was seeing double," Fishbein said in one of many interviews with me.

With the worsening of his symptoms, his doctor realized that they were not dealing with a sinus problem. "He said, 'I want you to see a neurosurgeon.' "

The twenty-nine-year-old graduate of Harvard University and Yale Medical School, together with his wife, had just moved into their first home three weeks earlier where they planned to raise their young daughter and their five-month-old son.

Six days after his first symptoms, the young physician was admitted to Montefiore Hospital in New York. A carotid arteriogram was performed. The procedure involved taking an x-ray of his carotid artery by injecting it with a radio-opaque dye. "It felt like an intense burning sensation, much like dysuria—the burning pain experienced on painful urination—except it was hot. It shot up my neck like a knife." The test indicated that there was a "space-occupying lesion" of undetermined origin in the rear of his brain on the right side.

Another test, a pneumo-encephlogram, was even more painful. According to Dr. Fishbein, "They pumped air into my head. It's like blowing up a football. I could barely sit up, but they kept telling me I had to remain upright. The procedure took three hours." That test confirmed the earlier findings. Based on the evidence from the two tests, surgery was performed to determine the exact nature of the swelling.

Surgery started at eight o'clock in the morning on November 12th of 1962. The surgeon, with his anesthetized patient lying face down, drilled four burr holes into the back of Fishbein's head. Using a surgical saw, the surgeon then detached the occipital bone from his skull.

With the bone pulled back, Dr. Wisoff, his neurosurgeon, now had access to Dr. Fishbein's exposed brain. He located the primitive, rapidly growing tumor in Fishbein's brain and cut out as much as he could safely. After the surgery was completed, Fishbein's occipital bone was repositioned and his head was closed up. Today, Dr. Fishbein refers to the surgical dents from the surgery in the back of his head as "finger holes" for a bowling ball.

Dr. Fishbein did not awaken from surgery until seven o'clock that evening and was unaware that surgery had taken place. Although much of the tumor was removed, parts of the deadly cell growth were located in places that were impossible to reach without killing him.

After the operation, microscopic slides of the tumor were examined by none other than Dr. Harry Zimmerman, a world-renowned physician who is considered to be the father of the field of neuropathology. Zimmerman determined that Fishbein had a "highly undifferentiated" cancerous tumor. A highly undifferentiated tumor is one made up of very young cells. Younger cells reproduce faster than more mature cells, which means the cancer will grow faster. A highly undifferentiated brain tumor is a little bit like having a pure stick of dynamite with a slow burning fuse. Physicians naturally equate such a diagnosis with a poor outcome for the patient.

Brain tumors often kill quickly due to the confined space inside the skull area. Even a slight growth of a tumor can affect a vital body function, such as the command center that controls a patient's ability to breathe. Because his tumor was especially malignant, Dr. Fishbein's doctors had estimated his survival time to be no more than two to four months.

Dr. Wisoff informed Fishbein's father, "I took out as much of the tumor as I could without killing him. He's in God's hands now." When asked if there were any chance of survival, Wisoff responded as truthfully as he could, "Not as far as I can tell."

Dr. Fishbein was not immediately made aware of the proper diagnosis. He was told that he would need radiation treatment for his "granuloma." The Yale medical school graduate knew something was terribly wrong:

"I responded, 'We don't radiate granulomas! What kind of granuloma is it? Tuberculosis? Fungal?' "

"The doctor looked kind of panicked, 'We're still studying it,' he said."

"I replied, 'Granulomas are infections, and we don't radiate infections!'"

Perplexed but desperate to start radiation, Fishbein's doctor told him the next day it was a virulent neoplasm. At that point, Dr. Fishbein's refusal to receive radiation quickly evaporated, and he agreed to have the treatment started, "as soon as possible." The regimen was quickly instituted, not for the purpose of a cure, but to help reduce the pain that was sure to occur from the pressure of the growing "rock" inside his head.

Upon Fishbein's urging, he was released from the hospital on November 30th. Although the medical consensus offered him no hope of survival, he immediately became a man with a mission to find a cure wherever it might be, "I didn't care if it was in China."

Although the post-operative swelling affected his memory, his coordination, and his fine motor control, he started a letter-writing campaign to every medical scientist he knew: "Sometimes I would write one word on top of another." Having attended Harvard and Yale, his mailing list included some of the brightest and most knowledgeable medical people in the world, including Professor George Wald, who would receive a Nobel prize the following year. According to Dr. Fishbein, Professor Wald responded, "Your letter makes me wish I knew more than I do."

In each of his letters he asked the recipients if they knew of any treatment for his condition. In each case, the return letters contained much sympathy and often included a promise to look further into the matter. None of the letters offered much hope, however, for the young family man's dire situation. Dr. Fishbein was determined to find help, nonetheless.

He worried as much about his soon-to-be-widowed wife and his young children. "I wouldn't see my children grow up. Who was going to take care of them?"

As he doggedly searched for an answer to the impossible, Fishbein came across an old mailing from Dr. Revici's Institute of Applied Biology (IAB) he had filed away years earlier. Seeing it reminded him of a conversation he had in a hospital cafeteria five or six years previously with Dr. Walter Leibling.

Dr. Leibling was a family physician who practiced a different specialty at each of several different hospitals in New York. Dr. Fishbein was highly impressed with Leibling's multiple specialties and had asked him if he could observe him for an entire day, just to see how he did it. Leibling consented to the unusual request. During lunch, Leibling let him in on a little secret and told Fishbein, "I know a doctor who melts tumors." Curiosity about Leibling's comment led Fishbein to write Revici's office regarding his work.

After receiving the mailing from Revici's office and looking it over, Fishbein filed it away and gave it little more thought.

Fishbein rediscovered the folder two weeks after his discharge from Montefiore Hospital. He went upstairs and immediately called Leibling. He informed his former acquaintance of his critical situation and asked him what he should do. According to Fishbein, Leibling said, "Go to him [Revici], don't argue with him, and follow what he tells you like a religion. Don't tell anyone and don't ask anybody else's opinion."

When he made the appointment to see Revici, Fishbein was asked to bring his records, so he called his doctor and asked that they be sent. The records never arrived. After a second unsuccessful attempt to obtain his records, Fishbein went to his doctor's office to pick them up personally. Fishbein explained to his doctor once again how time was of the essence, in that his estimated life expectancy was about two months.

His doctor refused to release Dr. Fishbein's records and said, "I'm not going to give them to you. As far as I'm concerned, you're a dead man." Shaken, Fishbein went out to the car where his wife was waiting for him. According to Fishbein, she said, "Let me try to speak to him."

She came back out to the car in tears. "He says he feels like he's talking to a dead man," she told him.

The other doctors he had dealt with were less cruel but no more hopeful. According to Fishbein they said things like, "There's no such thing [as a doctor who can melt tumors]. You're going to a charlatan. You're wasting your time."

When Dr. Fishbein arrived for his first appointment with Dr. Revici, the receptionist echoed Dr. Leibling's sentiments, "We find those who do the best are the one's who most closely follow the treatment."

During the first or second visit, Revici suggested he give John Heller, M.D., a call. At the time Dr. Heller was the head of Sloan-Kettering, which is perennially rated by U.S. News and World Report as the top cancer hospital in the United States. Revici told Fishbein he'd known Heller for ten years, and that Heller was interested in helping to arrange a study of Revici's method. (The study, known as the CAG, is discussed extensively in Part IV.)

Dr. Fishbein told Dr. Heller that he wanted to speak to him, "doctor to doctor," so he asked Heller about Dr. Revici. According to Dr. Fishbein, Heller told him, "I don't know how he does it, but people walk in there dead and walk out alive."

Intrigued by Heller's response, Fishbein asked him, "Would you recommend that I go to him?"

Dr. Heller answered, "Yes, I would."

When he asked Dr. Heller why Revici's method wasn't used at Sloan-Kettering, Fishbein says Heller replied, "I'd lose my job. I have to be careful around here. He's foreign, he's strange, and around here he's considered a quack."

Dr. Fishbein generally saw Revici three times a week for the first few months. After six months of treatment, Fishbein called Heller again to tell him that he was still alive and was doing better. Dr. Heller's response caught Dr. Fishbein off-guard: "What makes you think Revici's medicines had anything to do with your being better?" After the brief call, they never spoke again.

Fishbein gradually improved. A large part of Dr. Fishbein's short-term recovery came about as the post-surgical swelling in his brain receded. His walk steadied and his spirits soared. Meanwhile, the remnant tumor became entirely inactive.

Fishbein felt a debt of loyalty to Revici, so he volunteered his services at Dr. Revici's Trafalgar Hospital. The help was especially valued because the CAG study had just begun. He followed Dr. Revici on rounds and learned the rudiments of how to apply Revici's dualistic method. When Revici needed to travel outside the country, Fishbein would fill in by taking his place at the Institute.

Nonetheless, finding work became a bit of a challenge for Dr. Fishbein. "Nobody wanted to take a chance" on a doctor with brain cancer, Fishbein said. Despite assurances that his job would be waiting for him once he recovered his health, he lost his position at the Morrisania Hospital emergency room where he had worked three days a week prior to his illness. Five months after he began treatment with Revici and with no evidence of a tumor, this Yale-trained doctor and father of two needed to find work.

He had heard that Fordham Hospital in the Bronx needed a doctor for its emergency room. After the initial, positive interview, two weeks later the expected phone call came from a Dr. Kapp: "Doctor Fishbein, I don't understand. We want to hire you, but we got a phone call from downtown that says you're dying from cancer. You've got cancer of the brain. I don't understand. You looked fine to me."

He took a deep breath and told her he would come down to speak with her in person. In retelling the story, Fishbein said he didn't know what he would say to her when he arrived. But he went anyway and told Dr. Kapp about his illness, about his recovery, and about how his wife and children were depending on him. All he wanted, he said, "was a day's work for a day's pay. If I can't work, don't keep me here. I just want a chance to get back on my feet."

As Fishbein told his story, Dr. Kapp burst into tears, crying, "My Richard! My Richard!" Through her tears she managed to tell Fishbein a story about her own son. He had been a third-year medical student when he was diagnosed with Hodgkin's disease. "His friends were so cruel to him. They would say, 'Are you still here, Richard? Are you still holding on?' He held on for a while, and then he died."

Her eyes flooded with tears. She then told Dr. Fishbein how her husband had a heart attack at the funeral and died a week later. According to Fishbein, she looked at him and said, "Dr. Fishbein, when do you want to start?"

"She adopted me as her surrogate son."

As fate would have it, a similar occurrence would happen again almost three years later. Fishbein had a job interview with Mutual of New York (MONY) for the position of assistant medical director at the insurance company. When he told Dr. Lemke of MONY that he had brain cancer four years prior, Lemke informed Fishbein that he couldn't hire him due to his prior condition. In the course of their discussion Lemke revealed to Fishbein that his own twelve-year-old daughter previously had a cancer of the bone around her eye, known as Ewing's sarcoma.

Fishbein told Lemke that he hoped his daughter wouldn't be rejected by a college because some admissions panel might not want to waste an education on someone whose cancer might return.

Fishbein's answer caught Lemke unprepared. According to Dr. Fishbein, Lemke sat back for a few moments. "You know," he said, "I've never thought about it like that before. Let me see what I can do. Call me in a week." Fishbein was given the job.

Dr. Fishbein had been a talented violinist when he was in high school and undergraduate school. While attending Harvard, he had appeared on the popular television show Ted Mack's Amateur Hour and was invited back for a second appearance, which he declined. In fact, although he loved playing music, the demands of medical school would later cause the future physician to set aside the musical part of his life.

After his bout with cancer, Fishbein reacquainted himself with his first love and is now listed in the International Who's Who of Music. On one occasion, in 1972—nearly 10 years after his predicted death —Dr. Fishbein appeared with a couple of other musicians to perform at a party held by another physician. The gathering was attended by several more physicians who were aware of Fishbein's earlier brain tumor. Fishbein and the rest of the group played a four-hour program. "They just looked at me. They couldn't make any sense of it." They never asked him what had prompted his recovery, or anything else regarding his previous or present condition.

His recovery has also prompted him to write numerous clever and thought-provoking poems. They are often humorous poems that bend words from one meaning into the next while slipping a light philosophical notion into the mix.

As a final note, it should be mentioned that Revici's medicine never caused any harm to Dr. Fishbein or left him with any scars. In fact, Dr. Fishbein was able to return to work, to be a father to his children once again, and to rekindle his love of music as an accomplished violist, violinist and composer. To add a bit of icing to all of it, Dr. Fishbein is a newly married groom to boot.

And now, thirty-four years later, he is able to share with his new bride and with the world, the funny conversations he was able to enjoy with his children, thanks to Dr. Revici. That just might be a cure in the fullest sense of the word.

13

Eighteen Miracles

*"Whether you are a medical or a non-medical person, when
you hear the stories of these cases, when you see the x-rays of
bones eaten away by cancer and then returning to normal,
how can one but believe?... I hope we can get more medical
people to see the light and put his treatment into practice."*

DR. LOUIS E. BURNS, 1955

In April of 1995, *Parade Magazine* ran a story about an operation to
remove a brain tumor from a patient named Deborah Hubbard. Also
featured in the article was her physician from NYU Medical Center,
Patrick J. Kelly, M.D., who is considered by many to be one of the top
neurosurgeons in the country. The Parade article referred to Dr. Kelly
as "the father of computer assisted neurosurgery."

The popular *Parade Magazine* is no stranger to medical success stories and frequently acts as a public relations vehicle for new high-tech
treatments and medicines. From the perspective of the medical community, getting a story told in *Parade Magazine* is quite a coup.

Four months after the *Parade* article, the weekly magazine, *U.S. News and World Report*, featured a cover story about a sweet-looking seven-year-old boy named Matthew Anderson, who just had brain surgery. The cover photo grabbed onlookers' attention with a head shot of the smiling boy wearing an angry row of thick staples in his skull as a badge of courage. The headline on the cover boasted of "The medical miracle." The ensuing article told of Matthew's parents finding their medical savior when a Sunday school teacher passed along a copy of Dr. Ben Carson's autobiography entitled *Gifted Hands*.

It should be clear to anyone who watches television news or television-news magazines, or reads popular magazines, that anecdotal medical success stories are the life blood of maintaining public interest and support. The general public might not be aware that medical institutions and research centers actively cultivate the constant publicity they receive, and that the competition for media attention is quite stiff.

In general, Revici hasn't sought out attention among the lay community for his method. On one occasion he did present a number of interesting cases to the press. The occasion was a fund-raising effort for the newly purchased Beth David Hospital which was about to be renamed Trafalgar Hospital, a 177-bed facility which Revici would head for over two decades to treat desperately ill cancer patients. In 1955 Revici's Institute of Applied Biology (IAB) presented to its sponsors, members of the press and some medical people, some examples of the Institute's successes at that time. A fund-raising arm of the IAB, the Cancer Research and Hospital Foundation, announced its intention:

> For the purpose of observing the progress made by the Institute in the treatment of hopelessly advanced cancer cases, 18 patients selected from a larger group attended this conference. These included cancer of the stomach, bowel, breast, skin, brain, lymph nodes (Hodgkin's Disease), tongue, liver, kidney, ovary and thyroid. They were all considered beyond all help or hope.

In each case that was presented, the patient appeared on stage for a brief interview by Dr. Revici and by organizer and benefactor, James Van Alen. Mr. Van Alen was a successful businessman who became a strong supporter of Dr. Revici's research after asking his own physician, Dr. Louis E. Burns, to look into the Revici method. On the occasion of the presentation, Mr. Van Alen read from the letter he received from Dr. Burns:

> You requested that I look into Dr. Revici's treatment of cancer. This I did, and find it far beyond my wildest expectations.... His results are amazing.... They include cancer of the breast, prostate, skin cancer, melanoma — the highly malignant type that always kills – lung and bone cancer, the majority of these showing signs of retrogression. What a happy group of patients, too.... I must say it is the first time we have had a sound chemical approach or treatment for this dread disease.

Van Alen pointed out that each of the patients to be presented had previously had their cancer verified by a biopsy—performed not at the IAB—but by independent doctors at "many different hospitals." According to Van Alen, almost every person who was to take the stage should have already died from their cancer, at least according to the best prevailing evidence at the time.

A transcript was made of the event and published in a booklet entitled the "Report on the Revici Cancer Control." The cases were so remarkable that highlights of the patients' stories bear repeating here. In the booklet, the patients were referred to by their first name and last initial. For the sake of convenience, only their first names will be used here. The statements have been edited in some cases for the ease of the reader while attempting to maintain each speaker's original vernacular as much as possible.

Case History: Emma's right breast was removed in 1935. Eight years later [1943] she was found to have cancer in many of her bones. While under Revici's treatment her pain disappeared completely. Her bones, which had turned to jelly, "reconstituted themselves."

Emma: "Since I started on Revici's treatment, I have never lost any time from work except in the beginning when I was in the hospital. Since then I have continued to work steadily."

Case History: Francis contracted cancer of the tongue in 1942. The standard treatment is surgical removal of the tumor which causes a loss of part or all of the tongue. Cancer of the tongue is usually exquisitely painful. Under Revici's care the tumor gradually disappeared, and Francis remained well without treatment for thirteen years.

An M.D. from the audience: "This is the most persistent type of cancer, the most resistant to any type of treatment outside of surgery.... To me this method is new. I am in this field, and it's very stimulating. It will keep me awake at night.... You can't talk, you can't laugh, you can't eat, you can't do anything when you have cancer of the tongue."

Audience: "Do you consider this patient cured?"

Dr. Revici: "All we can say is that the lesion disappeared, and there has been no recurrence in the tongue during 13 years."

Case History: Melinda was a fifteen-month-old girl with cancer of the bowel that had spread to her lymph nodes. She was brought to Dr. Revici in 1948. She is now "attending school and she carries on all the usual activities of a child her age."

Dr. Revici: "We have a report of the operation: 'It is an inoperable tumor.' The pathological report showed a malignancy."

Melinda's Mother: "After she was operated on, they said she had two months to live, and the doctors back in Dayton did not know of anything that would help her."

Dr. Revici: "The tumor was not removed. The prognosis was certainly very bad, although it's difficult to say that it was a matter of two months. However, the child is now well after [seven] years."

Audience: "How is her general health?"

Melinda's Mother: "Very good."

Mr. Van Alen: "Does she play games and run around?"

Melinda's Mother: "She is active just like other little girls."

Mr. Van Alen: "Could you say that this tumor was not merely arrested, but actually disappeared?"

Dr. Revici: "We have reason to believe that is true. She came at the age of fifteen months, now she is eight-and-one-half-years old."

Case History: Robbie was brought to the Institute at the age of six in October of 1947 with many enlarged lymph nodes and a diagnosis of Hodgkin's disease. After ten months of treatment she returned home to Texas with only one small node in the neck.

Dr. Revici: "We asked several pathologists—I believe ten—to review the microscopic slides in order to see what their diagnosis would be, in view of the unusual evolution in this case after treatment. It was entirely confirmed by everyone as typical Hodgkin's disease.... Now there is no trace of the disease."

Case History: Benjamin came under Dr. Revici's care in January 1949 exactly one year after an exploratory operation revealed an inoperable cancer of the kidney. Six years later, "He has been symptom-free most of the time and continued to work as a truckman for various cleaning and bakery establishments. The tumor mass has not grown larger during this time. He has occasionally neglected to take medication, and at such times he tends to develop symptoms of pain and discomfort, and sometimes blood in the urine. When he resumes medication, these symptoms are controlled. There is no evidence of spread of the disease."

Benjamin: "I do a normal day's work. In fact, I went back to business since then, on the doctor's advice, and I'm doing what I've always done, quite energetic work. In other words, I deliver Arnold's bread and different items. It's quite strenuous. I serve seven or eight stores a day. I'm up at 3:30 in the morning and work until 12:00 or 1:00 o'clock."

Mr. Van Alen: "What is the life expectancy after a tumor like this is found to be inoperable?"

An M.D. from the audience: "I'd say from three to six months, possibly nine months. But the man is doing well after so many years, he feels well. That's the important thing."

Case History: After surgery in January of 1950 for his stomach cancer, Irving had lost 36 pounds. Narcotics were ineffective in relieving the pain. "He was admitted to various hospitals, but was discharged from each with the diagnosis of terminal cancer" which had spread to his chest.

After seeing Revici he responded excellently. His pain was relieved and "evidence of lung involvement slowly disappeared in serial x-rays. He has gained over 55 pounds."

Irving: "I was practically gone. My wife, son and daughter carried me in and sat me down in Revici's office."

Dr. Revici: "Because the metastases [spread] to the lung and liver, we were afraid to stop the medication. In some cases where we have stopped the medication there have been recurrences. It's extremely easy to take drops.... We intend to continue the treatment for a while."

Irving: "I came to Bellevue, and they didn't want me; at Kings County Hospital, they wouldn't even give me a bed."

Audience: "Why was that?"

Irving: "I guess they figured, what is the use of admitting him, just to lay there and die."

Case History: During surgery in February of 1951 Mae was found to have cancer that started in her ovaries and spread to her bowel, uterus, liver and throughout her abdomen. She underwent treatment with Revici while still at Lenox Hill Hospital. A large tumor that, "filled the entire lower abdomen disappeared, and she gained weight."

"[Mae] was entirely relieved of pain and returned to her usual activities. After two years, all evidence of disease had completely disappeared. The treatment was discontinued." However, in November 1953, the cancer became active once again. "Treatment was reinstituted and after six months, the abdominal masses had disappeared, and she was feeling fine."

Mae: "...my doctor explained it was just a swelling and in a year's time would disappear. But from what I understood later, he did not expect me to last a year. He expected me to last a few weeks, and that was the end of it."

Mae's husband: "I was in on the secret completely. The doctor said we hit a very bad case. She has a belly full of cancer. I asked him how long she would last, and he said, 'From what I saw 30 days, 60 days, maybe 90 days.'"

Audience: "The growth was not removed at the operation at Lenox

Hill Hospital?"

Dr. Revici: "Only a biopsy was done."

Dr. Burns: "I am convinced that no other method has offered so much medically....

"Whether you are a medical or a non-medical person, when you hear the stories of these cases, when you see the x-rays of bones eaten away by cancer and then returning to normal, how can one but believe?... I hope we can get more medical people to see the light and put his treatment into practice."

Case History: Dennis came to the Institute in March of 1952 with a deteriorating condition caused by an inoperable cancer of the stomach. He'd lost 50 pounds since he had first become ill and was experiencing loss of appetite, vomiting, nausea and abdominal pain. His progress under treatment was excellent. His symptoms were relieved, he regained his strength and weight back, and has been back at his old job as a construction foreman for nearly three years.

Dennis: "When I went in there [a nursing home], I couldn't eat a half-slice of toast, I couldn't drink milk, I couldn't eat Jell-O, nothing. The medicine Revici gave me put me on my feet again—when I came to Dr. Revici, I was crawling."

M.D. in the audience: "Here is the report from Brooklyn Doctors' Hospital. 'The [back] wall of the pancreas was involved with a [rapidly growing] mass, with glands near the liver, and along the aorta. Diagnosis: Advanced carcinoma of the stomach.'"

Dr. Revici: "Nothing could be done—the mass couldn't be removed."

Case History: For seven years Mary had developed a persistent ulceration around her left eye. Despite treatment with radiation, the tumor spread to a wider area. Several surgeons told her she would require a surgical procedure that would necessitate removal of her eye and the bones surrounding it. She refused the surgery, since she felt her appearance would have made it impossible for her to continue to obtain employment as a housekeeper. She began treatment with Revici on October 22, 1953. A biopsy of the ulcerated area was performed at Brooklyn Eye and Ear Hospital and revealed a recurrent carcinoma. Under Revici's care with lipids, Mary's ulcerated area healed and has since been covered by new, healthy tissue.

Mr. Van Alen: "Can you see with your left eye?"

Mary: "Yes, I can see better out of that eye now than I can from the other one."

Dr. Revici: "There has been no recurrence."

Case History: In June of 1954, Gis developed a sudden massive tumor in her bowel. By July it had spread to her liver. Part of the tumor was removed during bowel surgery, but the remaining tumor in her liver continued to cause her pain. Following a year of treatment at the IAB her pain disappeared, she gained weight and her enlarged liver returned to normal size. She had never been informed of her true condition, so her brother, a physician, presented her case.

Dr. V: "I've been a practicing physician since 1922. All of a sudden in June of 1954 my sister developed massive rectal bleeding. After surgery her doctors told me it was in the liver, and they couldn't touch it. When I asked what he could do with x-rays? he said, 'Nothing.' He had given her the death sentence.

"Revici told me she was doing all right, just to give it time. She started to gain weight soon after the treatment began. I think in less than two months she returned to work, had all her strength and all her normal weight plus three pounds. In this hot spell she never stopped work for one hour, in a shop that's not air conditioned, and her energy is marvelous."

Dr. Revici: "When this patient came to us her liver was enlarged and there was a mass like a tennis ball in her abdomen. It's gone and her liver is absolutely normal in size."

Case History: Leon had a history of numerous malignant tumors in his nose and on his face. They grew slowly and multiplied to the point where his appearance was very unsightly, and his job as a salesman was seriously endangered. With Revici's lipid treatment the tumors shrank.

When the medicine was reduced, however, they grew larger again.

Leon: "I went to the Institute and they gave me injections. In the first week it cleared up. They looked normal. I'd had a lot of others around my nose here and a lot of small spots coming out. The treatment cleared them all up. There was a time when I didn't have too much pep. Since coming here I feel better in general."

Case History: Alice developed the first of two lumps in her throat in the summer of 1953. A biopsy indicated cancer. Surgery could only remove some of the tumor. New masses invaded the surgical wound. With Revici's lipidic treatment the tumors shrank and disappeared.

Dr. Revici: "I haven't seen this patient in four months. She came down from her home in Canada by plane yesterday. How are you feeling?"

Alice: "I feel well now."

Dr. Revici: "She had a series of lumps, one big one here. It disappeared in less than a month. Do you feel any lumps now?"

Alice: "There is nothing now, not since I saw you in the Spring."

Case History: Twenty-four-year-old Nina had undergone a disfiguring surgery to remove a tumor from her cheek. The cancer grew back in two months. In April she was put on lipid therapy and received a small amount of x-ray therapy. "The rapid response of this rather resistant form of cancer to relatively small amounts of x-ray therapy was unexpectedly good. The administration of lipids has apparently improved the result to be expected from x-ray therapy in this patient."

Dr. Revici: "It was very painful."

Nina: "I have no pain now."

Dr. Revici: "You had pain before?"

Nina: "Sure, a lot of pain, yes. I am very much better now."

Case History: In March of 1954, ten-year-old Walter had the first of three brain operations. The tumor returned. The second surgery was performed in August. During a third operation in February, "only a piece of the tumor was removed." With Revici's lipidic treatment,

Walter's headaches and drowsiness went away, as did the swelling in his head. The involuntary movements of his head, extremities and body were also greatly reduced since the beginning of Revici's lipid treatment.

Dr. Revici: "What did the doctor tell you before you came to us."

Walter's Mother: "It was a only matter of time before he was going to die. They could not do anything more. I went to Columbia-Presbyterian and they wouldn't even look at me after I told them about the case. The doctors gave up on him. [Since coming here] they have done wonderfully with him. His nervous system has been wonderful, no reaction, no sleepiness and no more headaches."

Case History: Ten-year-old John was opened up in May of 1955, due to a hard abdominal mass. The surgeon determined that the mass was inoperable. A biopsy of the tissue performed at the time of the surgery proved the mass to be malignant. When John first arrived at Beth David Hospital, he had explosive diarrheal bowel movements, nausea and vomiting. In two months all his symptoms disappeared entirely. The abdominal mass could no longer be felt. He gained fifteen pounds.

Dr. Revici: "When he came to us his liver was very much enlarged. Today the patient is well enough to play baseball."

Audience: "What games did you play yesterday?"

John: "I played punch ball and soccer. Then we went fishing."

Van Alen: "What did they tell you at the hospital?"

John's Mother: "The chief of surgery said, "You have another son. Let him be a comfort to you. He also said nothing else could be done, he had the type that was resistant to x-ray."

Audience: "How did you hear of Revici?"

John's Mother: "Our private physician said, 'Why don't you take him to the Institute, because you can't just sit back and watch a wonderful boy die.' When we took him, he was very bad. He used to throw up all the time, and he slept all day. The diarrhea has stopped and everything is wonderful. I just look at him – well you just saw him. It was just wonderful."

Audience: "They said you should just take him home and keep him happy?"

John's Mother: "How could you keep him happy? When he came home he was thin, like caved in."

Van Alen: "This is one of those instances …it's hard to believe…just opened and closed?"

John's Mother: "Nothing was removed, and it was only twenty-minutes until they came and said nothing could be done."

Dr. Leonard Goldman, radiation oncologist: *"There is almost no spontaneous disappearance of cancer. I can't recall any case I have seen where there was a spontaneous disappearance of a tumor, and I've seen about ten-thousand cancer patients. There is always a reason for a tumor disappearing. They don't disappear spontaneously. There must be some chemical change that accounts for it."* (emphasis added)

Case History: Lydia, 27, had breast cancer that spread to her lymph and skin on both sides of her chest after breast surgery.

Dr. Revici: "The pain has disappeared. The visible tumors are reduced from twenty, to three or four. The remaining tumors are one-tenth their previous dimensions."

Dr. Burns: "I talked with this young lady this morning and we got along pretty well with my French and her Portuguese. She said she had very strong pains before, with great pain on the right side, and now she has none. She had about twenty lesions on her right side, and there is only one left now."

Case History: Janet, 33, suffered from swelling on her neck. X-rays showed the enlargement extended down into her chest. A biopsy indicated a malignancy. Lipidic therapy has reduced the neck mass almost entirely and the swelling in Janet's upper chest. It is planned to keep the patient on the lipids for a long time. This approach isn't possible with regular chemotherapy or with x-ray.

Dr. Revici: "She had a large mass, and that mass has disappeared in a month."

Case History: Albert, 45, had a malignant kidney that was removed, but the disease spread to several areas in his lungs. After several months of treatment the tumors stopped spreading and several of the masses had shrunk. Although Albert had almost given up on his business activities, he has since returned to them and is embarking on several new ventures as well.

Van Alen: "I think you got up to 27 holes of golf the last time I saw you."

Albert: "I consulted radiologists; I consulted surgeons. I went to different hospitals. All confirmed nothing could be done."

Audience: "When did you start these treatments?"

Albert: "December 2nd, 1954. In about two weeks I noticed that I seemed to be feeling better. Whereas before I had considerable aches and pains—today it's amazing—I don't even have a headache. I'm in a tournament right now, and I was matched with three friends of mine—all doctors. At the twelfth hole they were huffing and puffing all over the place, and I started to do better. They asked me where the heck I was getting all my energy."

After the presentation a physician in the audience asked if Dr. Revici was ready to, "impart this knowledge you've acquired." Revici answered in the affirmative, "I have always done so, since the beginning of this research. I know too little, but what I know I am very happy to tell to others."

The unidentified physician in the audience followed up on Revici's answer by saying, "I was told by friends connected with the American Cancer Society that Dr. Revici's methods aren't open to all who want to learn. When I met him, I realized how unfair that charge was."

A second physician, identified in the transcript as "Dr. Dutton" added, "I heartily concur that Dr. Revici is most willing to teach us anything he has. That has been my personal experience. I know it is a fact."

In the same "Report on the Revici Cancer Control" was included a 10-page paper Dr. Revici had presented to the Clinical Pathological Conference at Beth David Hospital on May 9th, 1955, in which he provided a brief summary of some of the major findings he had made in the area of cancer treatment. In the paper he discussed his findings on the progression of the malignant process and his ability to reverse that process by the administration of the appropriate lipids. He also discussed various testing procedures he developed to diagnose scientifically to which biological level a particular cancerous growth has progressed. The document is an excellent primer for any physician interested in learning more about Revici's method.

In the same "Report" was also included a two-page address given by Dr. Abraham Ravich two weeks prior to the presentation of that day's case histories of the 18 patients. Dr. Ravich called the transfer of Beth David Hospital to Revici's IAB to be, "one of the great turning points in the history of medicine and mankind."

In the same speech, Dr. Ravich mentioned the resistance they had encountered in some quarters. "We have repeatedly encountered opposition from certain individuals and groups who have mistakenly chosen to identify their interests with the maintenance of the status quo. But suffering humanity has accepted the status quo of cancer for too long already, and for this reason we ignore those who would delay us from our work and slow our progress."

Ravich then made a statement that has since become the missing ingredient in creating the widespread acceptance of the Revici Method. He noted that, "A larger measure of public support will be required."

If our hearts and minds are moved to consider the acounts of the two brain surgeries of Deborah Hubbard and Matthew Anderson, mentioned at the top of this chapter, as advances in medical treatment, we can be equally pleased by the stories of eighteen desperately sick men, women and children who have benefited from the medical advances of Revici's guided chemotherapy over 40 years ago.

14

Douglas Murphey: A 10-Year AIDS Victor

"There were people who came in who had AIDS who looked like they were at death's door. You came back a month or two later, and the difference in terms of their improvement was just incredible. He didn't rescue them all but, my Lord, he pulled a lot of people out."

ROBERT WILDEN, A REVICI PATIENT AND
NINE-YEAR VICTOR OVER CANCER OF THE JAW

The man on the other end of the 3,000-mile phone call sounded confident and relaxed. It hadn't always been that way. More than a decade earlier Doug Murphey would walk into his bathroom and be so disorientated he would have no idea why he was there. "Sometimes I would sit in a trance for hours." The neurological symptoms of his condition were only a part of his life-threatening condition.

His symptoms started with a parasite. In 1982 Doug's doctor gave him two powerful drugs that were supposed to eliminate the tiny intruders. Although the treatment might have killed the parasites, it left him with a persistent diarrhea.

As a gay man living in San Francisco, Doug had already seen a few of his friends suffer and die from AIDS. His own diarrhea continued for two years. "There I was in a body-based, very progressive psychology program. I understood the body-brain connection, and yet I was in complete denial. I could barely make it through class sometimes, the diarrhea was so bad."

By 1985 Doug's condition worsened. He experienced repeated cramping in his hands, feet and legs, "The pain was excruciating." Still, he couldn't bring himself to go to a doctor.

Finally in the early part of 1986 a friend convinced him to see Dr. Dwight McKee. A former associate of Dr. Revici, McKee was familiar with the principles of his method. He prescribed a nutritional therapy. After two weeks Doug's longstanding diarrhea cleared up.

But the overall progression of his illness continued. "I had a burning sensation on my skin, fatigue, and a lot of disorientation," Doug said. He had also lost thirty pounds.

Meanwhile, he had seen his mentoring professor, Judy Bell, struggling with a debilitatingly persistent viral condition that had been misdiagnosed as cancer. She had found out about Dr. Revici through a friend and went to see him in New York.

In July Doug's employer offered him a free trip to New York as a reward for the good job he had done in helping to rescue the company from collapse. Doug used the opportunity to visit Revici. He didn't have any medical records, nor had he ever had an HIV test done, so Revici instructed him to get the test and to come back to see him.

Although he complied by getting tested for HIV, he didn't return to Revici's office right away. He couldn't bring himself to even look at the test results. In fact, the results sat on his desk for a month before he finally opened the envelope. "I knew [before opening it] that all the test results were outside the normal range. I was numb." The lab results confirmed his fear; he was HIV-positive.

By September he couldn't cope with his symptoms any longer, so he returned to New York. Doug said he was emotionally on edge. "I asked him [Revici] how long I had. He said, 'Not long.' That really got my attention. Then he smiled and said, 'Maybe one hundred years.'"

Something stirred inside Doug. It was the hope he'd been looking for.

"Within the first hour [after treatment] the medicine completely eliminated my pain. I felt like a chalkboard that had just been erased, but not cleaned. The pain was gone, but I had a general feeling of not being clean." While he was in New York, Doug saw Revici every day, sometimes two or three times a day.

Around the sixth day he experienced a healing crisis. He had gone to the Metropolitan Museum with a friend. While there, he suddenly felt a withering feeling—he couldn't stand up. The pain came back in full force. His friend called Revici. Fortunately, the museum was near Revici's old 90th street office. Revici instructed him to come in right away. "He gave me five drops of a different medicine, and—boom, the pain was gone. That is what he was waiting for."

Later on, Doug would spend three months with Revici as an observing clinical psychologist. During that time he would notice that that type of reaction was not uncommon; patients would often have a worsening of their symptoms after five or six days of their first treatment. "I saw this happen time and time again with other patients."

The first three months back home would become his worst. His boss, who was also gay, fired him. "My boss asked me what was up, and then he told me he could no longer work with me." Ironically, his ex-boss would die of AIDS a few years later.

Meanwhile, echoes of his symptoms were coming back. He was constantly sleeping. "I was sleeping, just sleeping. [But] by Thanksgiving I was pretty much back on my feet."

From January through June he was taking a number of different substances, which is typical of Revici's treatment as a patient's condition changes. "By June, I was totally in the healthy range," according to his lab tests, Doug said. The doctors weren't prepared to accept the new results, "[They] thought there was a mess up in the laboratory." His doctor wasn't ready to believe that Revici's medicines had anything to do with his recovery and insisted that Doug come under his care. But Doug opted to stay with Revici's treatment.

"I wrote letters to the San Francisco AIDS Foundation, the San Francisco Health Department, the mayor and others." He heard "not a word" in response. Doug says that it was during the height of the AIDS hysteria in San Francisco, so apparently they weren't ready to believe anyone could get better. "I decided that wasn't about me."

By October of 1987 he was working with Donna Murray, Elizabeth Taylor's secretary, to put together an AIDS awareness week in the city under the auspices of the American Foundation for AIDS Research (AmFAR). During the middle of the week's programs, Suzy Tompkins, co-owner of ESPRIT, insisted that Doug drop what he was doing and come to her office.

When he got there, he was introduced to Teresa Crenshaw M.D., a member of President Ronald Reagan's AIDS Commission. Because of Crenshaw's influential position, Tompkins wanted her to meet an AIDS victor. Dr. Crenshaw declined to be interviewed for this book about her meeting with Murphey.

Soon after the AIDS awareness week, Doug was asked to come to New York to work with Revici. During the next three months, Dr. Revici, "made sure I saw him treat as many patients as possible. He seemed to be able to find the right moment with each patient to bring them out of their mind-set and into the frame of mind that would instill some hope in them." Doug says Revici never promised he would cure any patient, but found a different way with each one to provide a measure of hope.

Doug saw one patient whom Revici sent out to get more tests done before he would treat him. The desperately ill patient had apparently been a little difficult to deal with. When he returned for his second visit, his demeanor dramatically shifted. He burst into tears and told Dr. Revici how much he loved him. Revici pulled his eyes away from the weeping man as he contemplated the man's words. After a pregnant pause Revici looked back at the man, turning his head only slightly, and spoke with a smile, "Not as much as you will." According to Doug, Revici's remarks would have been the wrong thing to say to someone else, but for that man, the words provided the hope that he needed.

During the three months Doug observed patients. "I was seeing human disease and destruction at its worst. Yet, it was a continual reaffirmation of what was possible."

On one occasion a patient was too weak to get out of his car. As Doug tells the story:

> It was only a year earlier that I was sick with AIDS. I went out to the door with a wheelchair, but the cars at the curb were parked too closely together to fit the wheelchair through. So I went out into the street to the car door. Inside [the car] was a bag-of-bones of a man who might have weighed 80 pounds. I picked him up in my arms and carried him though a lobby of waiting people, directly into Revici's office. Revici gave the man an injection, and then I took him back out to the lobby where he was to wait for an hour before seeing Revici again. About an hour later a man came to Revici's office door and said, 'He's ready to see you.' The man, who only an hour before couldn't stand up, was standing at the door unassisted, and he walked into Revici's office.

Not every moment at Revici's office was as inspiring, however.

The window in front of Doug's desk faced the street. He noticed one morning that the city had put up 'no parking' signs in front of the office. At the time, Doug guessed that the city must have had some minor repair work to perform on the street.

According to Doug, between ten-thirty and eleven-o'clock that morning he observed that a "huge garbage truck" pulled into the no-parking-zone. Two men in white overalls and rubber gloves climbed down from the cab. They went to the back of the truck and "pulled out two trash cans." They began to pull syringes and needles out of the trash cans. A camera crew was behind them along with a couple of uniformed officials who said they were from the department of health. The health officials claimed that they had found the needles in Revici's curbside trash.

Revici came outside. He was furious, but he kept his wits. He invited the camera people into the office and showed them the three biohazard trash cans the office used for the disposing of needles and other dangerous materials. He also pointed out that it was not the office's regular trash day, so there was no reason for them to put any trash on the street, let alone hazardous materials.

A less dramatic but still disappointing occurrence took place in 1993. A congress of physicians from around the world who had been successful in treating AIDS patients met in Zurich, Switzerland to discuss their findings. Dr. Revici and Doug Murphey were among those invited to attend. As a condition for his helping to organize the event, Doug requested that a panel of long-term survivors be invited to tell their stories.

In 1993, as is true now, conventional medicine had nothing resembling an effective treatment for AIDS patients. In the U.S. the search for a cure for AIDS had a high priority both in federal dollars expended and in societal interest, as exhibited by the constant national and international news coverage of the topic. Considering the high level of interest in the subject of AIDS, a conference that discussed treatments that seemed to show benefit would normally be heavily covered by the U.S. news media.

The panel of long-term survivors was assembled. The physicians whose modalities had produced these long-term survivors also attended. Although the U.S. media had been given prior notice of the conference, none showed up to cover the event, according to Doug.

In the mid-eighties, Doug Murphey was about to become a statistic. Instead he has become an eloquent spokesperson and an example of the efficacy of Revici's method. For the past two years he has trained health professionals in the dynamics of helping patients and the families of those who are faced with life-threatening illnesses.

With himself and other AIDS patients, Doug found that the patients who improved the most with Revici's method were the ones who followed it the most closely. Doug saw a number of AIDS patients who went shopping from one practitioner to another in their quest to recover. "The idea was, if one thing is good, then more will be better." According to Doug, the ones who left Revici or who tried to mix his with other approaches, usually ended up getting sick again and dying.

Doug has not been immune to the many losses. He told me he had a large amount of fluid drained from around his heart. His body/mind-based psychology training led him to comment, "It's as though my heart was weeping for my friends." In our conversation he said, "Three died just last weekend."*

It doesn't have to be that way.

---

* Several months after our series of conversations, I was saddened to learn that Douglas had a recurrence of the fluid around his heart and died as a result. He will be missed.

15

Let a Smile Be Your Umbrella

"I think it will be tragic if what he has discovered isn't institutionalized in some way."

BOB WILDEN, PATIENT

At first glance Bob Wilden's story might not seem all that special. He didn't have any pain, just a little bit of a lopsidedness in one of his cheeks. But even that wasn't all that noticeable. He found out he had cancer in his jaw, so he explored his options. He chose to see Dr. Revici. He never had any chemotherapy or any other treatment, other than Revici's. The treatment with Revici took a fair amount of time before he could be declared free of his cancer, but eventually he became healthy once again. So, what's so special about Bob Wilden's story?

He still has his face.

Dr. Edward R. Mopsik, an oral surgeon with a practice in

Washington D.C., examined Bob and realized that the surgery that was needed to remove his tumor would cause a great deal of destruction to Bob's jaw, teeth and chewing muscles. Even then he wasn't so sure the surgery would do much good because the tumor was deeply embedded.

Dr. Mopsik provided Bob with the option of going to Sloan-Kettering. During his medical training, Mopsik had been exposed to some of the surgical marvels that had been performed there over the years. In a telephone interview, Dr. Mopsik told me about one of the old photographs he was shown. The picture was of a man whose waist was resting on a small wooden square with wheels attached to it. The man's legs, groin and buttocks had been surgically removed. That the man could still be alive after a surgery of that nature was a testament to the knife skills of the Sloan-Kettering surgeons who performed it.

Although Mopsik wasn't so sure he would want to perform that kind of a surgery if given the option, he was confident that Sloan-Kettering had some outstanding surgical people. If there was to be any hope for Bob, Sloan-Kettering was probably the place he would find it.

Meanwhile, Bob knew a woman who had been to Revici and who had survived about ten years before dying from a cancer that normally should have killed her in ten minutes. During that period she was able to work full time. What impressed Bob is that the woman wasn't always faithful about taking her medicine, yet Revici seemed to be able to bring her back to health periodically anyway. He decided if he was going to be in Manhattan, he would visit both Sloan-Kettering and Dr. Revici.

At Sloan-Kettering the surgeon, accompanied by another physician, stood behind a lectern as he explained what he would have to do. Bob said the surgeon was, "ticking off what he needed to do very matter-of-factly with no emotion. It was probably something he had done before and didn't much enjoy doing. I sat and listened to the two surgeons describe how they would operate on me."

Bob said they were going to, "saw through my jaw and teeth like a can of sardines. Part of it [the tumor] was accessible but part wasn't. It butted up next to my sinus. It wasn't clear what type of auxiliary damage would be done." (According to Mopsik, it would have certainly required the removal of certain jaw muscles and salivary glands.)

Bob let the doctor know that he was also going to explore the possibility of Dr. Revici's treatment. Bob said the doctor told him, "We don't have any problem with alternative treatment, but in your case I certainly wouldn't advise it."

After seeing Revici, Bob called the surgeon to let him know he had decided not to have the surgery. "The doctor said he wasn't real keen about that." So he asked him, "What do you think is going to happen?"

According to Bob, the doctor said, "I'm afraid you're going to call me back in two or three years, and the tumor is going to be all involved up in your eye."

That was in March of 1987. Since then Dr. Mopsik has told Bob, "What has happened to you is pretty incredible." Bob didn't say so, but I would guess that when he heard Dr. Mopsik's comment, he grinned.

When I spoke with Dr. Mopsik, he told me that his partner's wife was very sick with cancer. Mopsik wanted to get information on the studies Dr. Revici had published in France before the war, because his partner was French and was preparing to go to Paris. It was apparent to me that Dr. Mopsik had seen with his own eyes the results of Revici's method, and he was looking for a way to introduce the idea to his partner in a credible way from one scientist to another.

As we spoke, I told Dr. Mopsik that Dr. Revici's method wasn't very well accepted in the United States, and I mentioned that the practice of medicine here was "rather hierarchical." He responded, "You're too kind. That's putting it mildly."

16

Radiation, Recovery and Relapse

"After radiation burns, the body continues to produce
[abnormal fatty acids]. When these levels get too high,
a strong catabolic reaction occurs and death ensues."

Dr. Emanuel Revici, "Deleterious Effects of Radiation
Due to the Production of Trienic Conjugated Fatty Acids:
Theory, Diagnosis and Treatment," revised May 30, 1986

"Diagnostic methods have been described [by me]
to determine, even after the fact, which person suffers
from radiation burns.... For those with more serious
radiation burns, I have described a variety of agents
which will inactivate the continued production of [abnormal
fatty acids] and to neutralize those already produced."

Dr. Emanuel Revici, ibid.

Back in 1974, John Tucker said he used to be, "a 200-pound, year-around body builder, hang glider and scuba diver." Then he developed a tiny cancer, which was removed surgically. Along with the tumor his doctors removed 27 lymph nodes, "just to be safe."

He was then given 3,200 rads of radiation from his groin area to his sternum. John told me he was given 25 doses of radiation, but found out later that 20 sessions is the recommended maximum. He says it almost killed him, and he has the burn marks on his abdomen to prove it. John now calls the doctor who irradiated him "a charlatan." The radiation had caused an inflammation in his intestine which gradually became worse. "It was as if my gut had turned into leather," John said. After an exploratory surgery, a surgeon told John that he saw scar tissue in John's intestines as a result of the radiation he had received.

His digestive system slowly became less and less efficient, until he was finally unable to process any food at all. "It would just sit there, and it wouldn't move. His weight gradually dropped all the way down to 125 pounds. "I looked like one of the survivors from Auschwitz at the end of the war. My refrigerator was full of food, but I couldn't eat it. If I ate, I threw up. I was starving to death." By 1979 he had to quit his job as a tractor trailer operator with United Parcel Service.

"I couldn't do anything. I was used to going out and doing things. You can imagine the depression. I was ready to 'off' myself. It seemed like [it would have been] an act of euthanasia."

In a lecture entitled "The Influence of Irradiation Upon Unsaturated Fatty Acids" presented in London in July of 1950, Dr. Revici had described the underlying factors that caused the condition like the one John was experiencing. The subject of that lecture was the motivating reason for the United States Navy's earlier interest in Dr. Revici's participation in their nuclear program. Revici found that the effects of radiation poisoning would often worsen over time as more and more of the victim's fatty acids became abnormal. The effect of the radiation was often insidious because a small amount of damage would grow worse and worse over time. And once the amount of abnormal fatty acids reached a certain level, as measured by the oxalic acid index Revici devised, death was certain.

Fortunately for John, his mother and four sisters came to his aid during his suicidal crisis. They suggested he go to see Dr. Caroline Sperling, a psychologist. She had been a cancer patient of Revici's for four years. When she first went to see Revici, according to her own description, she had looked pregnant because so much fluid had accumulated in her belly from a far advanced case of breast cancer.* Dr.

---

* Although her original life expectancy was just a few months, she recovered and lived another nine years after first seeing Revici—her final bout apparently precipitated by a bad fall from a chair she was standing on in her office. Dr. Sperling was a cancer counselor in the Washington, D.C. area, and had sent many patients to Revici.

Sperling suggested that John see Dr. Revici.

Revici gave him a medication called "Twin 70," a twin formation compound. According to John:

"I swallowed this capsule. In two or three minutes it broke open and it felt like a cooling warmth, like menthol. The pain went from maybe a 'five' down to 'zero.' In two or three days it was like the inflammation was gone. It was like a miracle."

The improvement continued, "My life went back to almost normal, seeing friends and doing things. I'm a person of action. If I feel good, it's Katie bar the door."

As it happened, the Twin 70 became less effective as time passed. Finally, about a year later, the day arrived when the Twin 70 was no longer working. This type of occurrence happens with many of Revici's patients if their acid/alkaline balance flips from one side to the other. John also attributes the relapse to his tendency to overdo things physically. By this time John wasn't keeping in touch with Revici as often. Since he was on disability it was difficult for him to get to New York. Eventually, even walking a few blocks could trigger an episode of blockage or severe intestinal pain.

John's case helps to demonstrate why it is imperative that Revici's method needs to become standard practice, thereby making it available to anyone who might need it. His condition and the expense of travel made it impractical for John to see Revici when his condition flipped.

Unable to work, his limited means and poor health have prevented him from traveling to see Revici over the last several years. If Revici's method were widely available, John could go to a local doctor for continued care and have it paid for by his insurance.

A few years ago John had a large part of his intestines removed and has to depend almost entirely on "Total Parenteral Nutrition," which is nutrition by intravenous injection only.

Although he hasn't seen Revici in quite a while, he strongly believes Revici had the answer for his condition. His own experience with Twin 70 was so dramatic and distinct from his "Auschwitz years" he only wishes Revici's method could be available to everyone who needs it.

17

Joe Cassella: A One Per Center

*"Where are your chemotherapy survivors
if chemo is so great?"*

JOE CASSELLA, SEPTEMBER 1993

Joe is not a shy guy. He speaks his mind, but he doesn't need a lot of words to make his point. There was the time he stood up at a public hearing in 1993. But we're getting ahead of the story, because he wasn't supposed to live that long.

Around Thanksgiving of 1985 Joe found out that he had pancreatic cancer.

Pancreatic cancer is the same type of cancer that so quickly killed Michael Landon of *Little House on the Prairie*. Most people with this type of cancer don't last much longer than six months—which is one of the reasons why Dr. Seymour Brenner has selected it as one of the can-

163

cers to be treated in his study. The five-year survival rate for pancreatic cancer is one percent, according to the American Cancer Society.

An elevator installer, Joe weighed in at around 212 pounds until he became sick. Shortly thereafter his weight quickly dropped to around 170, he said.

Although he was scheduled for a complete course of chemotherapy, he took only one treatment. He had the chemo on a Friday, and by Sunday, "I was vomiting all day." It made his sugar level drop "way down." Joe already had mild diabetes. He figured that the chemo would put him into diabetic shock if he stuck with it, or just kill him outright. By February his doctor suggested he "go to Lourdes."

He started on Revici's lipid treatment in April of the same year and has been doing fine ever since, with his weight climbing back to about 195.

Joe is a loyal kind of guy, particularly to anyone who has saved his life. So, in September of 1993, when he heard there was going to be a Congressional hearing in Washington, D.C., and Revici's method was going to be one of the topics, he had to be present. He stood up and told his story. Then he sat down to hear what everyone else had to say.

As Joe tells it, "So, this lady doctor from NIH or somewhere gets up there and starts talking about chemotherapy like it was Holy Water or something. I was boiling. The place was full of people like me who'd gotten better seeing Revici and other alternative doctors. I couldn't take anymore, so I stood up and asked her, 'Where are your chemotherapy survivors if chemo is so great? They're not here because they're all dead.' They told me to sit down, that I'd already had my say."

Joe Cassella might be on to something. Nobody had to ask Joe to come to Washington, and no one paid his way. His involvement came as a natural response to his own healthy recovery after being told his best chance was a miracle at Lourdes.

If the medical world actually had an effective chemo treatment, radiation treatment or surgical technique, wouldn't people be talking about it? Wouldn't some of the beneficiaries of these methods have spontaneously come forward of their own accord by now? With the large number of people who have been treated with these techniques, wouldn't that army of supporters be quite large? After several decades of research and application of these methods, however, the absence of a spontaneous "Joe Cassella-type army" might have as much of a lesson in it as a stack of peer-review journals.

18

Brain Trust

*"Every surgeon has one case they can point to
that surpassed their best expectations."*

ROY SELBY, M.D., NEUROSURGEON AND CHAIRMAN EMERITUS
OF THE AMERICAN ASSOCIATION OF NEUROSURGERY

*"At this time, it seems that surgical techniques
have developed as far as is possible and further
improvements in prognosis and cure must await
contributions of other disciplines to eradicate this bane
of our specialty and our patients, the glioblastoma."*

ROY SELBY, M.D., JOURNAL OF NEURO-ONCOLOGY, 18:175–182, 1994

Brain cancers are nasty. The only "relief" they offer is the mercy delivered through their comas and quick deaths. Before those sad and unfortunate "positives" happen though, the head pains can be unbearable. Loss of bodily functions often accompanies the pain, and can make the life of the patient a frustrating and humiliating experience. People who were once active and vital can become totally dependent on others for their slightest need. In some cases behavior can become erratic.

Doctors don't like to call brain tumors "cancer" because the tumors don't metastasize. The blood-brain barrier keeps that from happening. Other than that difference, brain cancer does pretty much the same thing as other cancers—it lives and grows at the expense of the person who has it.

The blood-brain barrier often makes chemotherapy useless as a means of treating brain cancer because the chemo can damage the vital protection provided by the blood-brain barrier. The preferred modes of treatment are skull-dimpling surgery and radiation. Neither of those techniques is all that successful.

Surgery often causes injury to other brain centers, resulting in damage to various functions of the body, such as partial paralysis or the loss of bowel control. Nor does it provide much assurance that the tumor won't grow back. In fact, it almost always does because microscopic amounts of the tumor are usually left behind after surgery. This explains why not many people are seen walking around with the scars they acquired from brain surgeries. Their tumors come back, and they die.

There is something disagreeable about irradiating one's brain. In addition to striking the tumor, the radiation destroys any healthy brain tissue in its path. Oftentimes, radiation is used to reduce the patient's pain with no intent to cure the patient. It is called "palliative" treatment.

Finally, neither surgery nor radiation take into consideration the catabolic or anabolic condition of the patient.

In contrast to the scalpel and radiation, lipids slip harmlessly through the blood-brain barrier. They cause no scarring either internally or externally. Is it any wonder that brain cancer patients do well under Revici's care? Here are the stories of four more patients, each of whom had life expectancies of a few months. They have outlived those estimates by a combined total of more than 60 years.

At the age of twenty-four, while living in Atlanta, Ms Silver's first diagnosis was a Grade IV glioblastoma, which is probably the worst and deadliest form of brain cancer. It was determined that the tumor could not be removed surgically, according to Ms Silver's testimony ten years later at a Congressional hearing held by Rep. Guy Molinari of New York. A series of radiation sessions were prescribed. To clean out the dead tissue created by the radiation, surgery was performed by Dr. Joseph A. Ransohoff—a renowned NYU neurosurgeon—shortly thereafter. Joan testified, "At that point, they could not take all the tumor out. The tumor was too deep."

Ransohoff downgraded the original diagnosis to a Grade III glioma. A glioma can be a glioblastoma or any of a number of other brain cancers, possibly mixed with other cells. It is considered to be a slightly less malignant tumor.

Silver subsequently took chemo. "[T]hat lasted about two weeks. My white cells were going in the wrong direction." She decided to go to Mexico for Laetrile treatments. She stayed in Mexico for three weeks, but when she returned, "No one would inject me with it." Shortly thereafter she went to see Revici.

After a little more than a year of treatment with Revici, she returned to Atlanta where Dr. Alan Fleischer, the head of neurosurgery at Emory University did a CAT scan. "He walked into the room, and he said, 'This is incredible.' He could not understand how [my tumor] could disappear so quickly."

In a letter to Dr. Brenner dated November 11, 1987, nine years after the original diagnosis, Ransohoff downgraded the diagnosis once again saying it "could clearly have been even less aggressive" than a Grade III. In the same letter he also wrote, "Obviously, her response has been spectacular, and I am certainly interested in this follow-up."

In her testimony before Molinari, Silver also told of two other people who lived on the same street she did in New Jersey who had developed brain tumors within two years of her own. "My parents just kept saying, 'Please go to Dr. Revici.' None of them would. They both died within two months."

Jane Britt was just a teenager in 1982 when she was diagnosed with a Grade III, borderline Grade IV, astrocytoma, a cancer that resembles lumps in the brain. Ransohoff was her neurosurgeon as well. He removed part of the tumor, but it grew back.

Jane's mother, Dorothy, took her to Memorial Sloan-Kettering, where Dr. Jeffrey Allen examined her. Dorothy revealed at the Molinari hearing that the doctor told the family Jane's condition was so bad, "They couldn't even experiment on her."

The Britt family spent several hours at the hospital, "seeing all these children with all their hair lost and dying and screaming and yelling. I don't drink at all, but after we left that hospital, we went out and got drunk. We were so horrified."

Jane's tumor affected her body's ability to regulate its temperature. In the winter time she slept with the windows open, the air conditioner on, and with no sheets or blankets. She had headaches "at least three times a day," she testified. "It was nerves pulling in my head. I had so much pain I couldn't hold my head up, or my upper body up. A doctor said to me, 'What can I get you, my dear?' I told him, 'You can get me a gun. You can get me a gun, so I can blow my head off. I don't want to live any more.' "

Within four hours of her first treatment with Revici, her temperature returned to normal. "She was cold, because we took her in the car and she didn't have any coat on. Her headache went away until midnight. Jane's headaches gradually disappeared completely.

As with all of his patients, Revici instructed Mrs. Britt to monitor her daughter with a urine home-test and to call him, regardless of the hour, whenever changes occurred, either in the test or in Jane's condition.

Once, when Jane was in the hospital, Dorothy told Revici she couldn't call him back because she didn't have the money for the pay phone. "Call me collect, my dear," she testified. "I would call him at 3:00 [o'clock] in the morning, 5:00 [o'clock] in the morning."

Dorothy also told about a time when Revici's license had been suspended, "One time, Jane went for her medicine, and she walked into the office, and they had suspended his license, and it devastated my daughter."

Two days after her testimony, Dorothy wrote a letter to the Chancellor of the New York Board of Regents describing her daughter's recovery from her predicted certain death. "At one point a scan showed fifteen tumors in her head. When I took her to Dr. Revici six years ago, we had to carry her. She weighed 85 pounds. Now her vision has returned; she is working as a volunteer, and rides a bicycle."

Jane last visited Dr. Revici in 1994. She was doing fine and has since moved to Florida.

A third patient who had been treated by Dr. Ransohoff was also expected to die. Several months after he surgically removed 90% of her brain tumor, it suddenly grew back to its original size.

Prior to her illness, Joyce Eberhardt ran her own restaurant business and often worked 16- to 18-hour days. But Joyce, then 30-years old, began to slip away. Except for one hand, she couldn't move or talk. "She was slowly dying. The tumor was going to press on enough [nerve cells] to eventually close off her ability to breathe. She couldn't swallow, either," her husband, Andrew, told Rep. Molinari.

After her surgery and radiation treatments, Joyce was transferred to the Rusk Institute, a convalescent center affiliated with NYU, since there was little else that could be done for her. During her stay there, an attending physician advised her husband, "Take her home, love her, make her as happy and comfortable as you can, because she has only 6 to 8 weeks left." Instead of taking her home, her husband and her mother took Joyce directly to Revici's office.

Ironically, the person who told her and her family about Dr. Revici was a terminally ill roommate. She never went herself and subsequently died from an inoperable brain tumor.

Because of her nearly comatose condition at the time, Joyce doesn't remember many of the details regarding her recovery under Dr. Revici's care. But Andrew told the hearing room, "[Revici] put her on medication. We followed it to the letter. There were nights we stayed up all night giving her medication. She didn't respond immediately, but gradually she did. After about a year of his treatments, we went again and had a CAT scan and found, to our delight, that the tumor was dead."

Joyce and Andrew now estimate that her total medical bills prior to seeing Dr. Revici might have approached one million dollars. In contrast, the treatment from Revici was much less: $175 for the first office visit and $100-a-month fee for the frequent, sometimes daily, telephone calls to Revici, and $100 for subsequent office visits. At least once, Revici called her from Italy. When I interviewed her at her home, Joyce described Revici as, "A little Santa Claus."

Joyce also continued to see her neurosurgeon, Dr. Ransohoff, from time to time. She said that he once asked the medical students who were with him to leave the room when he saw her because he could not explain to the class why surgery was not indicated without also revealing her care by Dr. Revici and the results he had obtained.

Earlier, in a September of 1985 letter from Ransohoff to Joyce's personal physician, he refers to her "amazing recovery" and states an MRI "clearly suggests" her improvement could be attributed to radiation treatment given to her for seven weeks, two years earlier. Ransohoff claimed the "vascularity" of the tumor had been beneficially affected by the radiation. A tumor's vascularity helps determine its ability to grow.

Ransohoff's preliminary assessment is at odds with the fact that her tumor had grown back to its original size several months after the radiation treatment was stopped.

Over the next several years, Ransohoff would continue to use the terms "amazing recovery" and "amazing improvement" to describe Joyce's case. Ransohoff's letters never mention Revici's intervention which began in April of 1984.

Dr. Ransohoff has relocated to Florida in recent years. In a telephone interview, he informed me that these three patients were to be part of a review study to be completed by another physician at NYU. Unfortunately, he said, the records on Silver, Britt and Eberhardt were thrown out after he left.

Joyce's case illustrates the extreme caution many physicians exhibit in acknowledging to other physicians the beneficial effect of Revici's medications. It also highlights the fact that Revici's medicines cannot be given in hospitals. Trafalgar Hospital, which Revici had opened in 1955, closed its doors in 1978 due to financial problems. After its closing, patients could be seen on an outpatient basis only. It was not until Joyce was removed from the Rusk Institute that she could begin Revici's treatment. To this day, patients who require hospitalization are almost always cut off from Revici's medicines.

Joyce presently lives with her husband, Andrew, in New Jersey. She is cancer free.

The fourth member of our brain trust is Andrew Hamilton. His story begins in February of 1980. Always a bright and studious young man, this fifteen-year-old's grades suddenly dropped from A's and B's to C's and D's. "I remember my tenth-grade English teacher asking me if I was having problems at home." Shortly thereafter, Andrew was taken for a psychiatric exam at Sheppard-Pratt Hospital in Baltimore. The psychiatrist found nothing wrong with him mentally, so he suggested a physical evaluation. In March a lemon-size tumor embedded in the pituitary area of his brain was found on a CAT scan. Surgery could not remove it all, so radiation followed. "The radiation gave me a terribly sore throat," Andrew said.

After the radiation was completed, Andrew started receiving steroid treatment. "I was hungry and thirsty all the time." Every night he was allowed a milk shake made with skim milk to ease the soreness. His weight shot up from 135 to 220, all on a five-foot-five-inch frame. By July the tumor was growing at twice its previous rate, and his doctor told Andrew's parents their son would live only another two to four months.

Fifteen years later Andrew and his family would tell their story. We had gathered around the family's kitchen table with his mother and father. His younger brother, Floyd, joined in as he leaned against a kitchen counter. The entire family was excited about the possibility that Dr. Revici would finally be getting some of the recognition they felt he deserved.

During Andrew's July 1980 stay in the hospital, he asked his Dad if he was dying. "I just kept asking my father. I knew I was dying. I don't know how to explain it, but when you're dying, you know you're dying."

When Andrew spoke about his pain, he spoke with the horror of someone reliving the experience, "I was in such miserable pain the only thing I wanted to do was sleep, because when I slept, it was the only time I wasn't in pain. Your whole head feels like it has this big heavy bowling ball, and it's pushing its way out, and there's no way for it to get out."

Allan and Pierce Hamilton, Andrew's parents, were already strongly religious; this crisis made them even more so. They prayed daily and wrote their relatives and friends asking them to pray for an answer for their situation.

Meanwhile, Andrew's parents took him to see Dr. Shamim, a holistic physician in Laurel, Maryland. Dr. Shamim pulled a copy of Revici's book off the shelf and told his parents that Andrew's case was beyond his own expertise. He recommended that they seek Revici's help.

When he first saw Revici, Andrew was so weak he couldn't lift his right arm or his right leg, "I was three-quarters paralyzed on my right side." His younger brother, Floyd, provided his older brother with a great deal of help. He would carry Andrew when he needed to be moved around the house and would sometimes help Andrew clean himself.

Revici advised the Hamiltons that although Andrew's tumor was technically considered to be benign, it was a difficult one to treat, and that it might take several months before results might be seen. Under Revici's care, Andrew progressed slowly. His headaches diminished over a five-month period. A year after Revici's treatment began, Andrew walked into Revici's office under his own power.

His normally frugal parents were so excited about his recovery they bought him a motorcycle when he asked for one. He felt really proud that he could ride the bike and maintain its balance with both hands.

By November of that year he had a part-time job after school working in the kitchen of a retirement home. "I scrubbed the heavy pots by hand. There wasn't any grease in my pots when I was done. I could use both hands."

Andrew's first visit with Dr. Revici cost $50. It lasted an hour. The other visits were $30. During a visit to the Hamilton home, Allan Hamilton showed me 10 canceled checks totaling $320 – the entire cost of Andrew's treatment from Dr. Revici. The Hamilton's also donated $10 each time they were given a new medicine. "But that was not required," Allan said. In a little less than two years, Andrew no longer needed to see Dr. Revici. Since that time he periodically has a brain scan. The last one, like all the others, checked out fine. Unasked, the middle class family would later contribute $2,000 to Revici's legal defense fund in gratitude for what Revici had done for them.

Today Andrew works for the Social Security Administration.

19

To Be or Not To Be

"I want to have a baby."

"You haven't got a womb.
You can't have a baby if you haven't got a womb."

FROM MONTY PYTHON'S *LIFE OF BRIAN*

Professor Judy Bell had a womb, and she wanted to have a baby some day. In the Monty Python movie it was funny. In real life, Judy's doctor wanted to take her uterus out.

"I was getting a new virus or illness, it seemed, every day," Judy said. Her condition of daily illnesses continued for a few months or more. "Then I missed a period."

Her doctor ran some tests. Her prolactin reading came back "extremely high." Convinced she had cancer of the uterus, the doctor wanted to remove it. Unsure of the doctor's quick diagnosis, Judy had an MRI and a CAT scan done. Neither showed a tumor, but with her

175

high prolactin reading, her physician thought it was just a matter of time before the tumor would become visible. Exploratory surgery on her pituitary gland (which resides at the base of the brain) was also recommended. Judy was twenty-eight, and teaching psychology at Antioch West University where Douglas Murphey [Chapter 14] was a student.

One of the criticisms of Revici is that he cures people of cancer they don't have. The charge is made although almost every patient Revici sees has had a biopsy confirmed by others. In all cases, patients who haven't had biopsies are sent to get one prior to treatment, unless the patient adamantly refuses. According to Judy, when she saw Revici in 1982, he told her, "You, don't have cancer, you have a viral condition." It is perhaps ironic that if her first doctor had removed her uterus, he might have claimed that Judy Bell was cured of the uterine cancer she did not have. Fortunately for Judy, Revici did have some anti-viral medications.

Revici gave her three medications, "I was too anabolic. Within a day I stopped feeling sick. In the next two years I was sick only five days." Judy says that all of her subsequent Pap smears have been clear. Although her doctors still thought she might have a brain tumor, Judy's health has remained excellent ever since seeing Revici 13 years ago.

After having interviewed Judy by phone, I happened to meet her by chance at Revici's office in Manhattan. Residents of the West Coast, Judy and her husband were on an authors' tour promoting their new book *Love is for Life: creating lasting passion, trust and true partnership*. She looked beautiful, vibrant and healthy. She had just stopped by to say hello to her favorite doctor.

Her biological son, Kiva, is almost seven.

20

Climb Every Mountain

*"You know, it's a funny thing, about a half-hour after
I get my shot, I feel a drawing in my breast, on the lump,
and also, up on my neck I get another feeling the same way.
There's a little spot in my right breast that feels exactly the
same; in about a half-hour it pulls and draws."*

A PATIENT, NOW A 25-YEAR BREAST CANCER VICTOR, AS QUOTED BY HER BROTHER,
RAYMOND K. BROWN, M.D., AT A CONGRESSIONAL HEARING

You've got to love Sarah Siff—if you can keep up with her. This
sparkly-eyed, seventy-eight-year-old lady likes to go for daily five-mile
walks around mid-town Manhattan, Little Italy, Soho or wherever else
you'd like to go. Two summers ago she spent a couple of months hik-
ing in the hills of England and Europe.

About ten years ago her surgeon insisted he had to remove her
entire breast due to a cancerous growth he had found. She compro-
mised and let him perform a lumpectomy. Then her doctor recommended radiation. She refused and went to see Dr. Revici. According
to Sarah, when she went back to her first doctor, "He couldn't believe

that I'm okay." After examining her, he told her, "Excellent, [there's] nothing there," she says.

She can't say enough about Dr. Revici, "I don't know anyone who comes close to being like him. You just want to cuddle him like a teddy bear." She saw him on his 99th birthday. "He's a little more frail, but his mind is there. He talks to you."

She used to be able to get her treatments with Revici covered by Medicare, "but no longer."

When I last spoke to Sarah, she said she was not getting around as much since she broke her wrist a year ago. But in her next breath she told me about her all-day hikes up and down the carriage trials outside Bar Harbor, Maine in the Arcadia National Park. "When I'm there, I can walk all day and not be tired," she said. She went there not once, but twice this past summer. "There are lots of mountains and beautiful lakes, like Lake Sebago." She enjoyed seeing the seals and puffins around Bar Harbor as well.

When she's not stateside, she might be in Antarctica with a group of docile Chin Strap Penguins following her, or in the Galapagos Islands —two trips she has already made.

Sarah is dreaming of going to Tanzania for her next big trip.

21

Two Lung Cancer Victors

Lung cancer is a deadly business. The American Cancer Society statistics show that only a small percentage of people with the disease survive five years. Ask yourself—if that's true, where are they? Ask yourself if you know anyone who had lung cancer five years ago who is still alive. The typical lung cancer will migrate to the spine or the brain. First the patient is crippled, and then he dies.

Please let me introduce two people who have lived a total of twenty-eight years since they were diagnosed with lung cancer: Charlotte Louise and Norma Leonard. Both were patients of Dr. Revici, of course.

Charlotte Louise is a beautiful woman. If you saw her, you would never guess that she once had oat cell cancer, a really fast-growing disease that normally kills its victims within weeks or months of diagnosis.

When I first met her, I thought there had to be a mistake. In our phone conversations she had indicated her age. But the woman standing before me appeared to be fifteen to twenty years younger. Surely she couldn't be the same woman who had been told 17 years earlier that she would be dead in six months if she did not continue her chemo.

But she was.

According to Charlotte her troubles began in 1980. A bronchoscopy was performed. The tissue was abnormal and the doctor told her, "It looked like oat cell." The preliminary diagnosis was confirmed shortly thereafter. Prior to the confirmation, another tumor that was found on her ovary was removed.

After the surgery she was given three sessions of chemo to attack the oat cell tumor in her lung. It made her vomit constantly. "It was like a terrible flu to the hundredth degree," she said. While undergoing the chemo she had also started following a nutritional program based on metabolic typing, originally developed by William Kelley, D.D.S (no relation to author). Charlotte appeared to respond favorably to the chemo treatments, at least temporarily. Her doctor warned her, however, that her type of cancer "always comes back". But by that time she decided to switch her treatment to Dr. Revici and advised her oncologist of her plans.

According to Charlotte, the doctor was not happy with her decision, "If you don't continue the treatments, the cancer will return, and you will be dead in six months." During her office visit he also told her that she would be acting irresponsibly as a mother if she didn't continue the treatments. Charlotte asked that the physician not be identified since he is a highly respected physician in the community.

But the tumors never returned. She said that her doctor called her films, "Superbly normal. I was ecstatic." The doctor who warned her that she would die without treatment has since given credit to his own chemo for saving her life. Charlotte believes they both played a part in saving her life, but that she would have been dead long ago if she continued with the original chemo, "A little poison was good."

Charlotte continues to take care of her health through a variety of means including Buddhist chanting. Periodic checkups over the past 17 years indicate she is doing fine with absolutely no evidence of the existence of her previous illness.

A former stage and film actress, she now conducts workshops for patients with cancer.

According to Norma Leonard, her doctor likes her to come in for periodic exams—not because she has lung cancer anymore but because, "I'm the only survivor of my kind of cancer he's ever seen. It cheers him up."

It wasn't always that way. When she first learned of her lung condition, "Every morning in the shower, I would cry." The radiologist gave her 5,400 rads of radiation, a large amount by any standard. She developed a "blown vein" which prompted her to forego any more radiation therapy. "I couldn't give any more," she said.

She decided to make an appointment to see Revici.

Eleven years later, her husband says he can't keep her at home, "She is one of the busiest people I know." A retired special education teacher, she was elected to a four-year term on the Monteville, Connecticut Board of Education in 1993.

Norma is about to introduce a mentoring program wherein professional people in the community will visit the schools to talk with students about their work. She hopes to have a special program for the gifted and talented students in which CEO's and other successful members of the community will spend time with the high school students. She is also active with the Monteville Youth Services Bureau working with crafts and organizing youth programs.

Norma's activities provide yet another example of the difference between current cancer treatments and Dr. Revici's method of treatment. Norma is pleased that she was lucky enough to find Revici.

She wishes people would at least have the option that she had. "I've learned until people are ready for something, there's little use in pushing. I used to traipse the Revici stuff to my friends. None ever used it, and all of them have died."

22

Some Results with 372 Patients

In the foreword of this book Dr. Seymour Brenner has written briefly about a proposed study to test Revici's method on patients with incurable cancers. He has also remarked to me that, after seeing tens of thousands of cancer patients and never seeing a case of spontaneous remission, that if one out of the hundred patients in the study were cured, it would be significant evidence of the efficacy of Revici's method. Of course, if two or three were cured, it would mean that much more.

A study was conducted on Dr. Revici's method by Dr. Edoardo Pacelli, in Naples, Italy. Like Brenner's proposed study, only terminally ill patients were used. The condition of the patients was so poor, in fact, that the average life expectancy of its participants was less than 90 days. All of the patients suffered from wasting away (cachexia). Although Dr. Pacelli makes no mention of it in his report, it can be assumed that many of the patients also suffered from the debilitating effects of treatments received prior to entering the study group. In April of 1984, Pacelli prepared a preliminary report of his findings in summary form on the six most common locations of cancer treated in the study.

Pacelli evaluated a number of factors, including the average survival time of the patients, their pain levels, quality of life, and weight loss. Other factors were also taken into account. For example, the lung cancer patients were evaluated regarding coughing with blood, and intestinal cancer patients were monitored regarding fevers. A total of 372 cases were included in the report. Not one of them was considered to be curable.

Pacelli and his staff treated 186 lung cancer patients. A number of remarkable improvements were achieved despite the extent of their illness. For example, nearly half were afflicted with metastases—either in the bone or in the brain.

The coughing up of blood disappeared in three-fourths of the 102 lung cancer patients who had suffered from this condition previously. Upon entry into the study, 60% of the lung cancer patients suffered from pain that could not be controlled by medication. With treatment, 80% of the patients either had no pain at all, or their pain was reducible with medication. Three-fourths of the group gained back most of the weight they had lost in the three months prior to treatment.

The lung patients initially had an average life expectancy of 80 days. Average survival at the study's close for the lung cancer participants was 172 days. 45% of the patients were still alive at the time of the report, so the actual average survival time was understated in the report. In addition to the positive effect on life extension, the quality-of-life index for the group doubled from 35 to 70 (out of a possible 100.)

Fifty-seven intestinal cancers were seen. Forty of them had multiple metastases. Their average life expectancy was a mere 60 days for these patients when they entered the study. By the end of the study, the average intestinal cancer patient had lived 245 days. Twenty-one of the intestinal cancer patients were still alive when the results of the study were written, so once again, the average survival rate of the patients was understated.

Three-fourths of the intestinal cancer patients had severe pain upon entering treatment, but for nearly two-thirds of that group, pain either disappeared or was significantly reduced. While 65% of these patients had fevers at the start of their treatment, fevers disappeared for 80% of them. According to the report, "Abdominal fluid regressed in 70%" of the intestinal cases treated. The quality-of-life index for the group climbed from 30 to 80.

Fifty-three patients with Stage IV breast cancer were treated. Upon entry into the study, 92% of the breast cancer patients had pain that could not be relieved by medication. Of that number, 80% of them found their pain to be either eliminated or reduced during treatment with Revici's medications.

The average survival for the breast cancer patients had doubled by the close of the study. Average survival time was 180 days and counting, with 12 of the patients still alive at the time the report was written. The average quality-of-life index also more than doubled for these patients, increasing from a poor 25 to a score of 60.

The average survival time for uterine cancer patients tripled to 270 days and counting with nine of 27 patients still alive when the report was prepared. Originally their condition was so poor that their average life expectancy was a mere 90 days. Pain was reduced in 71% of the uterine cancer patients. In addition to living longer, the quality of life of the average patient doubled from 35 to 70.

The patients with liver cancer started the study with an average life expectancy of a mere 60 days. With Revici's medicines the liver patients' average survival time was 233 days and counting with 42% of them still alive at the close of the study.

Of the patients, 20% regained 100% of the weight they had lost in the three months prior to treatment. The other 80% gained back an average of 70% of their weight loss during the same period. Almost half of the patients had pain that could not be controlled by medication upon entering the study. Of the entire group, 65% experienced pain reduction. Once again, quality of life improved significantly from 25 to 70 for the average patient.

Prior to the study, 20 of the 23 stomach cancer patients had either relapsed or had metastases. They began the study with an average life expectancy of 75 days. These patients had lived an average of 265 days and counting with nine of the patients still alive when the report was written. Of the stomach cancer patients, 75% suffered from intractable pain accompanied by vomiting whenever they tried to eat. In 90% of those cases their pain was "strongly attenuated."

Sixteen of the stomach cancer patients suffered from night fevers when they entered the study. Every case of fever was eliminated. Almost all of the stomach cancer patients regained an average of 80% of the weight they had lost in the three months prior to entering the study. Only 4% of the stomach cancer patients continued to lose weight.

In a test of any experimental cancer drug, almost any one of the above findings would be considered worthwhile, particularly if the drug caused no toxic side effects. The sum of all the findings noted by Pacelli from extremely sick patients with multiple tumor sites and other very severe problems provides a useful window into the value of Revici's medicines. Compared to the results reported with standard chemotherapy drugs, radiation and surgery, the results achieved by Pacelli are nothing short of phenomenal.

The fact that this study was conducted in Europe by someone other than Revici also diminishes the argument that the results Revici has achieved with his patients are due merely to their response to Revici's kind and caring manner. In fact, the argument that Revici's results are psychologically induced unfairly discredits the many kind and caring oncologists who have been unable to match Revici's results. Kindness and caring are important factors in all medical care, but the type of results achieved by Revici or Pacelli would be much more widespread if caring and kindness were the only necessary ingredients to a patient's recovery.

In his 1955 paper, "The Control of Cancer with Lipids," Dr. Revici wrote:

> [I]t is our feeling that the method of cancer chemotherapy that we are utilizing ought to be applied in cases of cancer as soon as possible after the diagnosis has been determined. Generally we believe that it is preferable to apply the method before, rather than after the disease has reached the systemic phase.

Common sense tells us Dr. Pacelli's success would have been that much greater if his patient population had been treated in the early stages of their cancer. The idea that Revici's method should be reserved for those who can no longer be helped by standard treatments might very well be a backward approach in cancer treatment. As Carolina Stamu, M.D., has said of Revici's method, "It's not alternative medicine—it's real medicine."

23

"I Forgot How Much Pain There Is"

"'Spontaneous remission' means that the disappearance of an illness happened by chance, a one-in-a-million occurrence."

GERALD EPSTEIN, M.D.
HEALING INTO IMMORTALITY

Dr. Lawrence LeShan has written a dozen books* discussing the correlations between certain psychological states and cancer. In fact, his studies are recognized by many as pioneering work in that area. Supported by independent grants not connected to Trafalgar Hospital or the IAB, LeShan spent twelve years conducting research with patients at Trafalgar. He undertook further studies at other hospitals, including Walter Reed Army Medical Center.

---

* Dr. LeShan's books include "Cancer as a Turning Point," "Einstein's Space and Van Gogh's Sky," "The Medium The Mystic and the Physicist," and "You Can Fight For Your Life."

During those years he had many opportunities to observe Revici at work with patients. As he told the New York Congressman, Guy Molinari:

> I have never seen a more dedicated physician. I have never known before a physician who told every charge nurse in the hospital that if he was needed at any time, by any patient, he should be called, and to my personal knowledge if he was called at two, three or four in the morning, he was always there within twenty minutes.

When I interviewed Dr. LeShan at his Manhattan apartment, he stressed how Revici made every effort to save each patient. "So often in cancer a patient is completely abandoned medically. [At Trafalgar] no patient was ever given up on. No patient was ever given palliative treatment. Every patient was fought for every inch of the way."

LeShan became habituated to the relatively pain-free cancer patients at Trafalgar. After four or five years, he went to Walter Reed to collect data for a research paper. "I forgot how much pain there is. I was absolutely shocked by the amount of pain that was there, at a very good research hospital. They were screaming in the halls. They were lying on the floor tearing up sheets. With Revici, which were really all terminal cases, there was really very little pain."

One Christmas weekend, LeShan spent a late evening with a British oncologist going over the files of discharged and deceased patients. According to the physician's analysis, many patients who should have died recovered completely. LeShan recalled, "[Revici] certainly got some results. My own best estimate is that among the *absolutely* hopeless patients, where the expected recovery rate was one-in-ten-thousand, one-in-ten would walk out in good shape with long-term remission."

LeShan says the criticism Revici attracted came because, "He started something too early. His file cabinets were full of papers he couldn't get published."

According to LeShan, despite the critics, Revici tried to teach his method to anyone who would listen. The attitude of most physicians, according to LeShan, was fear. "[Their attitude was] I don't want to be tied up with Revici and have my name muddied up, and the rest of it. I saw this."

One story LeShan related paints a picture of the depth of resistance that exists among some of Revici's peers. While visiting a former lung cancer patient of Revici's who had been hospitalized due to a heart attack, LeShan ran into a physician. On the way out of the hospital, he was stopped by the doctor. As LeShan relates:

> He said, "Oh you're from Revici's office. I know all about Dr. Revici. I know a charlatan when I see one. But I'll tell you this, I'm not one of those people who simply accepts what people say. I've read his book, and I've examined his medications. His book is semantic nonsense and his medications are garbage. But there's one thing about the guy that puzzles me. That bastard has the highest rate of spontaneous remissions in the country."

24

No More Migraines

Beginning in 1950, Bernard Welt, M.D., an ear, nose and throat specialist, wrote a series of extensive articles regarding Revici's method—not for treating cancer, but for a number of other conditions. The articles were published in a peer-review magazine called *Otolaryngology*. Two of them concerned the condition of dizziness known as vertigo. The other two articles dealt with head and neck pain and the post-operative pains resulting from nasal and throat surgery.

In each of the four studies, Dr. Welt's research confirmed Revici's theory of the causes and mechanisms of those conditions in most cases. In fact, Welt found that Revici's dualistic approach and his lipidic medicines provided superior results over what could be accomplished with standard treatments in many cases. In one article Welt wrote, "The results of... these studies confirmed the findings of Revici about the biochemical processes taking place in pathological tissues.... These concepts present a new approach to the study [of vertigo and head and neck pain.]"

Much like the results Revici achieved with cancer, Welt found that treatment with Revici's medications were often dramatically effective for his patients, "I was able to correct the abnormal metabolism in a majority of cases." These patients had previously been universally unsuccessful in finding a medical solution to their problems.

As mentioned earlier regarding migraine patients, Dr. Welt was able to help every patient in his study. Suspicious of the results claimed by Dr. Welt, Revici challenged him on it. Revici said he told Welt, "Nothing exists in medicine one hundred percent." According to Revici's testimony before Molinari, Welt laughed and said, "I am sorry that today I have not one case yet of migraine not responding to this treatment."

Patients in Welt's studies who exhibited no catabolic or anabolic imbalance derived no benefit from the Revici-based lipidic treatment, a finding that would indicate Revici's method was helpful with pathologically based conditions but not useful for head and neck problems caused by structural misalignments.

Despite the success of Revici and others in treating patients with lipidic medicines for a variety of conditions, his method and medications have never caught on with mainstream medicine. The logical question to that situation is, "How can that be?"

Welt's studies were apparently overlooked by the specialists in his field. It appears that dramatic news of success in the treatment of ear, nose and throat illnesses could not break through the consciousness of the American medical profession. Quite possibly this is because there was no underlying mechanism assisting the medical profession in taking the information to the next step. For example, there were no pharmaceutical companies behind Welt's research. Also, because the medications did not have FDA approval, other physicians would have little or no way to implement Welt's findings in their own practices.

By the time of Welt's groundbreaking reports, medical research in the U.S. reached a stage where only the findings of major research institutions with the backing of multi-billion-dollar pharmaceutical companies had a chance of being implemented. Today, midsize biotech research firms, often working with the major pharmaceutical companies, also play a role. However, the basic situation remains unchanged. Solutions for this serious deficiency are discussed in Chapter 34 of this book.

Modern science sometimes scoffs at the idea that one system of medicine could prove to be beneficial for so many seemingly unrelated illnesses. In fact, the mere suggestion of the possibility often brings an instant vision of medicine men selling potions in brown bottles from the back of horse-drawn wagons. Yet the impressive results achieved by Drs. Revici, Pacelli, LaBurt, Sher, August, and Welt for a variety of conditions would indicate that premise needs to be revisited and revised.

Today, enough people die from cancer each year in the U.S. to equal the number of names on nine Vietnam War memorials. That war produced a huge outcry, with many people believing that there were many unnecessary deaths. Is it possible that the war against cancer, officially declared in 1971 by President Nixon, has also allowed much unneeded suffering and many unnecessary deaths? The next section will provide a behind-the-scenes look at some of the events that help to answer the question, "If Revici's method and medicines are so effective, why aren't they being used by everyone?"

PART IV

HIS FOES

25

"A Mexican Treatment for
Cancer—A Warning"

---

*"When **truly improved methods for the treatment
of cancer** are found, it seems self evident these
will quickly find wide application to all victims
of cancer without the advertising used to promote
the sale of cancer nostrums." (emphasis added)*

JOURNAL OF THE AMERICAN MEDICAL ASSOCIATION (JAMA)
COUNCIL ON PHARMACY AND CHEMISTRY, JANUARY 8, 1949

How could it be, if Revici has found "truly improved methods for the treatment of cancer," that those methods have not received wide acceptance, as indicated by the words of the JAMA Council above? Revici certainly hasn't advertised his "nostrums" in the pages of JAMA —or anywhere else, for that matter. In fact, his lack of advertising might place him in a category apart from the many pharmaceutical houses whose ads for cancer drugs and pain killers are found within the pages of JAMA on a weekly basis.

Just the same, in a less complicated world, the statement by the JAMA Council would very likely be true—a true cancer cure would "quickly find wide application to all victims of cancer." In that kind of world, if Revici had found a cure, it would be nearly impossible to keep the news from spreading.

In fact, that's exactly what happened. The word was spread by physicians who had seen with their own eyes what Revici's medications could do. Those physicians came from some of the most highly respected cancer treatment centers in the United States. They notified leading cancer researchers and sent patients to Revici's hospital which was then located in Mexico City. Some of those patients spread the word even further.

And then suddenly, the good news stopped.

The story starts when Revici arrived in Mexico in 1941. As mentioned before, he and his family had arrived on an overcrowded ship filled with some of the leading government officials from the Republic of Spain and a few of the top scientists from the European community. Revici arrived in Mexico with letters of introduction dating from his days in Paris. The letters reflected the respect with which Revici was regarded and also point out that he was already on a fruitful path in the treatment of cancer and other maladies.

For example, Dr. Leroux, a renowned researcher and professor of pathologic anatomy at the Faculty of Medicine in Paris, stated:

> Dr. Revici has been working in my laboratory for two years.... It is vital that his research be continued without interruption, for the results obtained by Dr. Revici open a multiplicity of new paths to research of all kinds, particularly in the field of cancer.

No less ringing were the words of Dr. Chifoliau, Honored Member of Hospitals of Paris and a member of the Academy of Surgery of France:

> On several occasions, in cases of patients afflicted with grave surgical conditions, I requested the aid of Dr. Revici, who willingly applied to our patients the results of his laboratory research. The results obtained in the most hopeless of cases were always the amelioration of pain, and quite often the progressive disappear-

ance of large tumors. Dr. Revici's research must be continued and fostered, and may change the therapy of tumors completely.

Dr. Chifoliau's remarks regarding Revici's ability to shrink large tumors and eliminate pain in grave cases stands in stark contrast to what would be published later in JAMA on three separate occasions.

Soon after Revici and his family arrived in Mexico City, his good friends, Gaston and Nenette Merry, joined them and helped finance the establishment of a new research clinic named the Instituto de Biologia Applicada (IBA).

As Revici would later write, the IBA:

> ...consisted of a clinic for outpatients, a hospital with all modern equipment, a clinical laboratory, a research department with eight laboratories, and a section for experimental research on animals. The staff... numbered fifteen physicians and chemists in addition to a personnel of sixty which included nurses, helpers, and order-lies. The records were kept in Spanish.... We were fortunate in interesting several eminent physicians, surgeons and scientists who were also refugees in Mexico City.

Although the patients paid a fee for their hospitalization, they were not charged for the treatments or for the medications used.

By the end of 1943 a Wilmington, Delaware banker, Thomas E. Brittingham Jr., became interested in Revici's work. Brittingham's father had been one of the founders of the McArdle Memorial Laboratory for Cancer Research at the University of Wisconsin. Brittingham, Jr. was furthering his father's interest in cancer research when Merry probably sent word to him of the activities of the Institute, according to writer Marcus Cohen.

Before long, doctors from McArdle and from the M. D. Anderson Foundation for Cancer Research in Houston, Texas came to visit Revici at the IBA.

On September 11, 1944, C. A. Calhoun, M.D., of the M. D. Anderson Foundation wrote of his experiences to the director, Dr. E. W. Bertner. In his letter Dr. Calhoun described the dramatic results he had seen during his stay there. For example, he told of a patient who was bedridden and in considerable pain due to extensive bone involvement. As a result of treatment the patient gained ten pounds, walked six to ten blocks a day and was out of pain.

Calhoun wrote:

> [McArdle] sent and paid the expenses of ten patients suffering from cancer.... [S]ixty per cent of these patients have benefited and the rest have died.... [B]ut the thing that impressed me more than anything is the fact that every patient in this institution is free of, or practically free of pain without the use of narcotics. In my opinion, if he has nothing else, this ability to relieve intractable pain is a great contribution.

Dr. Calhoun's comments that Revici's compounds almost universally eliminate the cancer patient's pain is consistent with the compelling testimony of Dr. Lawrence LeShan, presented in an earlier chapter.

According to Dr. Calhoun, one patient's lip became, "completely healed and looked quite normal." Regarding another patient, Calhoun wrote, "[A neck] tumor which had been the size of a lemon had completely disappeared." Prior to admission, a third patient had been, "screaming with pain for the last several weeks, and after forty-eight hours was having very little pain and feeling much better."

Six weeks after his first letter, Dr. Calhoun wrote to Dr. Bertner again and relayed more of his observations regarding the achievements at Revici's Institute. He described a variety of cancers that were helped, "I saw at least eight patients who are apparently cured." Calhoun's letter described the eight cases, including the case of a patient who regained the ability to walk normally after suffering from a spinal chord tumor that had caused the paralysis of both his legs. Another case that impressed Calhoun was a nasty tumor of the thigh bone, "which was apparently cured."

Calhoun went on to say that Dr. Lowell S. Goin from Los Angeles was also, "very much impressed with Dr. Revici's work and feels, as I do, that Dr. Revici is very sincere, and that his work and results seem promising enough to be more thoroughly investigated and continued..." Dr. Goin, an officer in the American Radiological Society, was yet another highly regarded cancer specialist who had heard about Revici's work and had come to see the results for himself.

Dr. Goin told Dr. Revici he was so impressed that he had written glowing letters to Cushman Haagensen, M.D., chief of cancer research at Columbia University; to Cornelius Rhoads, Ph.D., head of Sloan-Kettering Memorial Cancer Center in New York; and to a Dr. Pendergrast in Philadelphia.

By mid-December of 1944, Brittingham wrote to Donald C. Bell, M.D., in an attempt to convince him to become a one-year observer of the Institute.

On one occasion in Brittingham's presence, Revici performed a demonstration of the principles behind his method to an audience of several doctors including Dr. Bertner and Dudley Jackson, M.D., who was an officer in the Texas Cancer Society.

Dr. Revici prepared two glasses of water each of which contained an alkaline solution. He asked the patient to select one to drink, and had Dr. Jackson drink the other. The patient was known to be on the acidic side and had been experiencing considerable pain that morning. Within fifteen minutes of drinking the alkaline solution her pain went away. Meanwhile, Dr. Jackson noticed no difference in the way he felt as a result of drinking the same solution.

As a second experiment, Revici prepared two more glasses of a solution, only this time they were both acidic. Once again, he asked the patient to choose one of the glasses. Dr. Jackson drank the contents of the other glass. One eyewitness reported, "We saw her go from no pain to severe pain," during a fifteen minute period. Once again, Dr. Jackson felt no effects from his acid drink.

Dr. Revici then asked Bertner which alkaline lipid preparation he should use to eliminate the woman's pain. Dr. Bertner's selection was given to the woman by injection. The woman was then able to get out of bed by herself, something she had been unable to do for two months.

Revici then performed the same experiment with a patient who was diagnosed as having an alkaline pain pattern. This time it was the acid solution that made the patient feel better, while the alkaline drink caused him to feel worse. Once again, neither drink had any effect on Dr. Jackson. The exercise proved to be a dramatic way to demonstrate Revici's theory of dualism in pathology.

After describing Revici's repeated performances of this exercise with other patients to remove pain within minutes, Brittingham wrote the following:

> This pain work is universal amongst the patients and, as I see it, is certainly worth all the investigation, even with no other gambles....We did see a good many impressive cases from the cancer end.... There was a cancer of the femur [thigh bone] where the leg was back to normal size, and the x-ray showed the progress. All the doctors there agreed that the only kind of cancerous femurs they knew were those that had killed the patients in great agony....

Of the previously mentioned spinal tumor, Brittingham wrote, "Dr. Goin did a fluoroscope on her and watched the black material which he put in her spine run freely up and down her backbone," which indicated that the spinal tumor was no longer present.

In the same letter he spoke about a situation which, looking back, provides a possible clue to the later abysmal treatment Revici would receive from several of these doctors:

> To our group he [Revici] was 100% in the open. Absolutely nothing was held back, and as an outsider, I thought our group was quite insulting to him at times. If I had been in his shoes, I'm afraid I would have thrown some of our doctors out.

Five weeks later in mid-January, Dr. Goin wrote in a letter to Gaston Merry that he had treated two of his own patients in Los Angeles using Revici's method:

> Dr. Revici will be interested to know that I am treating a severe radiation injury.... Pain which had been severe, ceased entirely.... I was also able to control the pain of a terminal pelvic carcinoma with phosphoric acid...

On one occasion Dr. Goin's enthusiasm for the method led him to ask Revici if he could explain the results to some visiting doctors himself. Because his own English was poor, Revici was more than happy to let Goin proceed. During the rounds Goin presented several x-rays he had taken himself which demonstrated the disappearance of tumors in a number of different cases.

According to a notarized affidavit signed by Revici, during the next several months, his institute received numerous inquiries:

> ...not only from Texas and Wisconsin but from all over the United States. We would receive many communications from physicians, relatives and patients who wanted to know about the 'cancer cure.' They had heard about it, they said, from the physicians who had seen the 'cure' when they visited the Institute and studied the cases.

Throughout all this time Revici made no attempt on his own to advertise a cure or even to indicate to the public that he had some success with his method of treatment. To the contrary, he gave all the visiting U.S. doctors a handout—Revici was unsure of his spoken English—which said in part, "We consider our contribution only as a beginning. The results obtained thus far... show that we are on the right road, and nothing more...."

One would think that the doctors who had written as favorably as they had, and spread the word about Revici's method within the United States, would not turn their backs on him. Yet, on August 18, 1945, without prior notification to Revici either from the authors or from JAMA, a letter appeared in the Journal of the American Medical Association which indicates that nine of the visiting doctors did just that.

The contents of the letter in the Correspondence column matched its ominous all-caps headline in bold print:

A MEXICAN TREATMENT FOR CANCER—A WARNING

The letter would be the first of many assaults during the ensuing decades against Dr. Revici's approach in the treatment of cancer. It was signed by Drs. Bertner, Calhoun and Goin, along with six others. The majority of the doctors had seen for themselves the dramatic results Revici was obtaining by the application of his method.

One exception was Chauncey D. Leake, Ph.D., the Dean of the School of Medicine at the University of Texas. His only visit lasted some twenty to thirty minutes and consisted of a conversation between himself, Dr. Revici and Harold Rusch, M.D., who headed the McArdle Memorial Foundation for Cancer Research. It was Leake who had circulated the JAMA letter among the others and who had requested that they sign it.

Fellow signatory Rusch had been so impressed after seeing the results at the Institute that he had arranged for the previously mentioned trip made by the ten Wisconsin patients. He had justified the effort and expense because he believed the McArdle Foundation would be conducting further research based on Revici's work at the Wisconsin center.

The JAMA letter placed a negative cast on nearly every aspect of Revici's work. In the letter the authors attributed improvements in the patients due solely to Revici's,

> ...courteous and considerate bedside manner. We think he makes his patients feel better by virtue of his personality. There is no positive evidence that he or his associates are successful by their peculiar methods in interrupting the usual course of a malignant process.

As to the compounds themselves, the signers referred to the medications as "various glandular and tissue brews" and stated, "No positive evidence exists to indicate the value of these preparations in treating malignancy."

In addition to the thoroughly negative report about his treatment, they also criticized Revici's record keeping, referring to it as, "A characteristic but unfortunate aspect..." The letter then concluded with the following: "It is concluded that little benefit may result from cancer patients going to Mexico City for this new 'treatment.' " At that time the Journal was fond of placing in quotation marks treatments it deemed to be of questionable value or outright quackery. The same use of quotation marks by the authors would not have been lost on the medical readership.

Revici was stunned.

Years later in 1955 Revici would write a forty-one page response that included 100 pages of exhibits to substantiate his counterpoints. Using correspondence from the doctors in which they elaborated on the positive results they had witnessed, Revici responded to each and every statement made in the letter.

In regard to a charge of inadequate record keeping, Revici wrote, in part:

> This also represents a flagrant distortion of the truth. Each patient had a very complete record with daily observations written-in by the resident. They had daily analysis of two samples of urine, to determine the pH, specific gravity, chlorides and oxidized trypto-phan. Additional analysis for sodium, potassium and phosphorous were carried on for months on daily urine specimens. Except for special cases with daily blood analysis, all the patients had a week-ly C.B.C. [complete blood count]. Many had serial analysis of the blood lipids; and E.K.G. were often taken as part of the research.

Revici then proceeded to name several other tests and studies that were carried out "when necessary" as well as the use of a large Zeiss micro-photography camera. Revici also pointed out, "All the records were kept in Spanish, but a few were condensed and translated into English, and were at the disposal of all the signers of the letter."

The JAMA correspondence also faulted Revici's scientific approach:

> The theoretical basis for the methods of treatment are extraordi-nary. While they make use of scientific concepts, they are not in accord in any way with established biochemical or pathological considerations.

The letter in JAMA appeared to contradict what Dr. Rusch had said in a December 21, 1943 letter to Brittingham, when he wrote, "My visit with Dr. Revici was very worthwhile, and I am enthusiastic about some of his ideas. I must state, however, that most of his work is of a fundamental scientific nature."

In his 1955 written response, Revici also included a letter that was addressed to Dr. George Dick, chief of the Department of Medicine at the University of Chicago, from Gustave Freeman, M.D., a major in the U.S. Army on leave from an assistant professorship of medicine at the University of Chicago during the country's participation in World War II. In his letter, Freeman mentions that Dr. Goin and Dr. Jackson both sent patients to the IBA. (This is further substantiated by a letter that Jackson wrote to Revici in 1947 in which he relates the continued progress of a patient he had originally sent to Revici.)

In Freeman's letter to Professor Dick he went on to say:

> Naturally I've been most hesitant in believing what I saw.... I would not be inclined ordinarily to make any such proposals to you if I did not feel there was merit in the work... particularly when one considers the vast amount of research in the field of tumors with a few basic gains, and is worthy at least of a trial.

The letter was part of an effort by Dr. Freeman to have Dr. Dick extend an invitation to Dr. Revici to continue his work at the University of Chicago. In a recent interview, a cautious Dr. Freeman played down his favorable impression by saying that Revici's work was unproven and needed to be further examined. It is unlikely, however, that an invitation to the University of Chicago would have been extended to a foreign physician under those uncertain circumstances, without some evidence of success.

One interesting sidelight to the JAMA letter signers is brought to light in a letter from Merry to Dr. Freeman. He mentioned that Dr. Rusch was a co-author of a study published by *Cancer Research* that was practically a duplication of Revici's previous research published in France. In the letter Merry points out that Revici told Rusch all about it while Rusch took copious notes. Merry noted that Rusch gave no credit to Revici and used different terminology, perhaps in an attempt to disguise its source.

Another of the signers of the letter published by JAMA who deserves a special mention is Dr. R. T. Cooksey. Cooksey was a physician affiliated with McArdle. During a short visit to the IBA, he was introduced to a patient whose tumor of the neck was visible externally. Cooksey came back a month later and saw the patient to be much improved and wandering the halls. The once visible tumor had disappeared. The patient spoke English, so Cooksey was able to speak with him.

According to Revici's affidavit, Cooksey "expressed his amazement that the lesion was clinically healed, the tumor having disappeared." Cooksey asked if he could have the "before treatment" and "after treatment" photographs of the patient. At the time of his request, he told Dr. Revici and the patient that, "This case alone would be enough evidence in favor of the method."

When Brittingham later asked for the photographs to be returned to Revici at his request, Dr. Cooksey wrote, "I have been unable to find the photographs." Cooksey then went on to say that he hoped Revici would be able, "to do great things."

It's rather clear that the doctors visiting from the U.S. witnessed for themselves a startlingly new and improved way to treat cancer. Many of the letters that were written express in rather specific terms the positive results they saw at the IBA.

That the visiting U.S. doctors spread the word in a manner that caused numerous people to contact Revici is consistent with their own positive response to the Revici method. Dr. Goin's successful use of the method in his own practice provides yet another indication that Revici's method had merit. Furthermore, Cooksey's response to Brittingham's letter lends weight to Revici's account of Cooksey's favorable reaction to what he had seen at the IBA.

In short, the doctors' own behavior and words stand in stark contrast to their signing of the letter which appeared in JAMA. The turnaround was so strange, one might wonder how and why it happened.

In a situation like this there is a tendency to ask the victim why the perpetrators have done what they have done. Of course, Revici had only met Dr. Leake on one occasion and was not privy to his motivations. Revici guessed that Cornelius Rhoads of Sloan-Kettering may have been behind the letter, due both to his friendship with Leake and to his all-consuming desire to find a cure for cancer at his own institution. On more than one occasion Rhoads had said that if a cure for cancer were to be found, it would be discovered at Sloan-Kettering. Thus, the motive of competition is a possibility.

As late as 1949 the Journal of the American Medical Association's Council on Pharmacy and Chemistry wrote that chemotherapy was still an experimental therapy for cancer:

> Many promising discoveries… have been made which offer hope some day drug therapy may become an important measure, but until further research has been completed, the use of drugs must, for all practical purposes, be regarded as still in the experimental stages.

One staunch proponent of chemotherapy was Dr. Rhoads. He had previously worked with the U.S. Army on chemical warfare. From that work he introduced the idea that mustard gas might have application in the treatment of cancer. Based on the JAMA council's statement regarding chemotherapy, it is clear that Revici was ahead of Rhoads and others in chemotherapy research.

Ralph Moss Ph.D., author of *The Cancer Industry* and a former assistant director at Sloan-Kettering, cites a speech made by Rhoads in which he predicts a financial pot of gold for chemotherapy. Moss also notes that Rhoads had stated on more than one occasion that if a cure for cancer were to be discovered, it would be found at Sloan-Kettering.

Regardless of the JAMA letter, Revici continued his tireless schedule. He decided to accept the advice of friends who suggested he not stir up additional trouble for himself by sticking his neck out and taking on the powerful Journal or the letter writers by replying to the original correspondence. It is difficult to say what would have happened if he had fought back. As we shall see in the next chapter, the Journal might not have been receptive to a response from him, had he chosen to answer the letter. In any case, the Journal wasn't finished with Dr. Revici.

26

JAMA and the Romanian Immigrant

"It never happened."

Dr. Gustave Freeman, M.D., referring to an incident
contained in a report regarding Dr. Revici
in the Journal of the American Medical Association

As damaging as the 1945 letter might have been to Revici's medical reputation, it paled in comparison to the next step taken by the editors of JAMA less than four years later.

To understand the gravity of JAMA's follow-up action in 1949, one should first understand what it means to be a peer-review journal. To be "peer-reviewed" means that before an article is published in a scientific journal, it is supposed to be reviewed and scrutinized by other experts in the scientific community as to the article's accuracy. This process usually takes several months. The idea behind the peer-review process is that it ensures that no statement of purported fact is made without evaluation by other experts in the field. The reader of a peer-review journal places a higher level of trust in its articles for that reason.

On January 8, 1949, an article by JAMA's Council on Pharmacy and Chemistry appeared with the heading "Report of the Council" and the italicized statement:

"The Council has authorized publication of the following report."

—Austin Smith, M.D., *Secretary*

With that lead the average doctor would certainly have been led to believe that JAMA had made a special effort to examine and verify the facts of its report, and that it was a report of special significance.

Under the category of "FRAUDS AND FABLES" appeared a description of Revici's method that lacked almost entirely any semblance of accuracy. In fact, it summarized the false charges of the 1945 letter discussed previously. Instead of attempting to verify any of the information published in the 1945 "Mexican Treatment" letter, the Council chose to repeat some of its unsubstantiated claims.

The first paragraph concerning Dr. Revici began oddly, "Emanuel Revici, said to be a refugee physician from Roumania..." At the time Dr. Revici was a member in good standing in the AMA. JAMA is the lead journal of the AMA. Yet, JAMA declined to use the honorific of "Dr." before his name or the identifier of 'M.D.' after it. Its description of Revici seemed to imply that they were not sure if he was a licensed physician.

In 1949, the average JAMA reader was sophisticated enough to know that a refugee from war-torn Europe was probably Jewish. In an interview, Roy Selby, M.D., the highly regarded chairman emeritus of the American Association of Neurosurgeons, and a recognized medical historian, told this author that there was a great deal of prejudice against non-German Jews by members of the medical profession at that time.

Clearly, mentioning a doctor's heritage was not and is not the normal practice for scientific and medical journals, unless the article is referring to a study regarding a possible genetic condition. By describing Revici in that manner, JAMA failed to meet its usual high standards for fairness.

The Journal also referred to Revici's "treatment" by putting the word in quotation marks throughout the article and referred to Revici himself as "this person."

The article suggested that Revici fattened up his patients by giving them fatty acids: "His 'treatment' consists essentially of the administration of fatty acids by mouth and by injection under the skin, to induce a gain in weight." The article then went on to compare Revici's administration of fatty acids with the force-feeding of patients.

As Revici himself would point out, JAMA's fatty acid notion provided a true indication of the Council's lack of interest in objectivity or accuracy. The quantity of fatty acids used by Revici were measured in amounts almost too small to fatten a rat.

As disparaging and prejudicial as the rest of the comments were, there was one statement in particular that stood out beyond the others. The JAMA Council claimed the following:

> Subsequently, Revici spent a few months at the University of Chicago, where he was given the opportunity to demonstrate his method, with the result that in 52 patients with cancer, no favorable effects could be attributed to his form of therapy.

The charge was a damning indictment of Revici's method. Subscribers — that is, the medical community — would have been thoroughly convinced that Revici's method was worthless, because the Journal's Council had examined written reports of the application of Revici's method with 52 patients and found it utterly wanting.

It would appear that Revici's only recourse at that time would have been to argue that perhaps JAMA's Council on Pharmacy and Chemistry had overlooked some benefit of his treatment among the 52 patients.

But Revici couldn't make that argument. He couldn't make that argument because *he never treated a single one of those patients.* Nor did anyone else implement his method in the treatment of 52 patients. The JAMA statement was entirely and utterly false.

In 1946, at the strong urging of Dr. Freeman, Dr. Revici was invited to the University of Chicago (UC) by George Dick, M.D., chief of the Department of Medicine at the university. But within one or two weeks after Revici arrived at the university, Dr. Dick retired. Whatever support Revici might have had was cut off. He was not granted any hospital privileges. According to Dr. Freeman, who returned to UC at the time of Revici's arrival, there was a great deal of competition at UC within the medical research community. A new chairman at the school was expected to take the research in a different direction. Whatever the reason, Revici was not granted hospital privileges and was unable to treat a single patient at UC's Billings Hospital.

A small number of patients followed Revici from Mexico to Chicago and were treated by him privately on an outpatient basis. At least two of those patients continued to improve. In fact, two of the patients— who were among the 18 patients featured in Chapter 13—followed Revici not only to Chicago, but to New York, and continued to do well when Revici wrote his 1955 affidavit. Had JAMA been referring to Revici's private patients—which numbered far fewer than 52—surely they would have been required to include those two patients.

The AMA was already aware of Revici's inability to practice at UC because Dr. Freeman had sent a four-page letter to them in 1947 in which he explained that due to personnel shifts at UC, Revici had no facilities and was merely a guest of UC. The letter was handed over to B. O. Halling, the acting director of the AMA's Bureau of Investigation, who informed Dr. Freeman that the letter would be kept on file for future reference.

In reaction to the JAMA broadside, Revici responded with a fifteen page line-by-line devastating rebuttal of the "Mexican Treatment" letter and the JAMA Council article. It was addressed to JAMA Editor, Morris Fishbein, M.D. (no relation to Dr. Robert Fishbein.)

In return Dr. Morris Fishbein sent back a response. He told Revici and his associate, Dr. Abraham Ravich, that if they didn't sign-off on his own draft of a letter for the Correspondence column of the Journal, he would,

...submit the entire material to the Council on Pharmacy and Chemistry. They, in turn, would find it necessary to reply to statements from you which seem to be in effect an attack on the Council.

Fishbein, himself, was an influential member of that Council.

Of course, M. Fishbein's remarks could be construed in a number of ways. For the best interpretation it might be useful to look at other remarks M. Fishbein has made regarding alternative cancer therapies. For many years M. Fishbein placed himself at the forefront of the attack against those therapies.

In April of 1964 he gave a speech before the International College of Surgeons Hall of Fame which was later published in the Winter 1965 edition of *Perspectives in Biology and Medicine.* In his speech, entitled the "History of Cancer Quackery," M. Fishbein detailed his activities in eliminating "quackery" to the best of his ability.

As part of that speech, he elucidated some of the methods he used to destroy anyone who attempted to sue JAMA for its written statements regarding various cancer cures. In addition to commanding greater financial resources, M. Fishbein, in his role as editor of JAMA, also apparently enlisted the Internal Revenue Service to help harass the plaintiffs involved in lawsuits against the Journal. According to his own boasting, JAMA apparently had contacts at the IRS who would attend court proceedings at its behest.

In the written edition of his speech, M. Fishbein claimed:

> Needless to say, Koch [a physician who developed his own treatment protocol for cancer] never sued for slander or libel. Perhaps he had discovered that *every* person who had sued the American Medical Association following an expose had shortly thereafter gone out of business, frequently broke because of lawyers fees *and the attendance in court of the representatives of the Internal Revenue Service. (emphasis added)*

Whether or not his bragging about the IRS being at the beck and call of a private organization is accurate, M. Fishbein's statement indicates that the remarks he made to Revici were to be taken seriously, especially by a refugee physician who had once escaped certain death at the hands of Hitler's fascism.

In his speech, M. Fishbein included Dr. Revici by name. He mentioned in passing that fifteen physicians from California visited Revici in Mexico, "[They] were so impressed that they wrote a letter to *The Journal of the American Medical Association* highly commending his work." That letter never appeared in the Journal.

We also know from Fishbein's remarks that he had a copy of Revici's 1961 book and had at least flipped through it: "More recently Dr. Revici sent me a great tome replete with pictures and arguments for his method of treatment, which he calls 'biologically guided chemotherapy.'" Directly following that statement, M. Fishbein repeated a negative summary opinion made by the American Cancer Society in 1961 regarding the Revici Method. That ACS opinion will be examined in the next chapter.

In his final remarks, Fishbein painted Revici and others in graphic phrasing reminiscent of an Edgar Allan Poe short story:

> Of all the ghouls who feed on the bodies of the dead and dying, the cancer quacks are the most heartless. Heaven speed the day when the advance of medical science against cancer, most dreaded of diseases, will deprive these ghouls of the sad soil on which they nourish themselves.

That is the Dr. Morris Fishbein with whom Dr. Revici pleaded to reexamine the record more closely on his behalf.

Six months after the Council's attack on Revici, a letter signed by Dr. Abraham Ravich on behalf of Revici's Institute of Applied Biology finally did appear in JAMA. None of the evidence from Revici's fifteen page refutation was allowed to appear, however. Nor did JAMA run an apology for their prejudicial and fanciful statements, including the 52 "ghosts".

What was unknown to JAMA was that in 1947 the Federal Bureau of Investigation had conducted a comprehensive background check on Revici to obtain top-secret security clearance for him stemming from its interest in having Revici perform medical research in support of its nuclear weapons program.

While Revici was still in Mexico, he had carried out extensive research in the treatment of radiation burns with results that were extremely promising. It was the same research that indirectly had enabled Dr. Goin to successfully treat a radiation burn patient of his own. Of course, a security clearance was necessary if Dr. Revici was to participate in a military program regarding nuclear weapons. As part of that investigation, an FBI agent checked out Revici's activities while at the University of Chicago.

A Freedom of Information Act request filed in the mid-1980's revealed the results of that background investigation on Revici. The FBI agent wrote in his report that there was no evidence of Revici treating any patients at UC's Billings Hospital.

The FBI agent's report was consistent with a letter written by Dr. Freeman in which he said, "It never happened." Recently, Freeman emphatically confirmed his written statement in a telephone interview from his residence in Palo Alto, California, "It certainly did not." Freeman was in a perfect position to know since he was the one who had paved the way for Revici's invitation to the university and worked along side him during Revici's short stay at UC.

Freemen did attempt to treat two patients of his own who were very close to death. His goal was to see if the medication would help reduce the pain they were experiencing in their final days and hours. Both patients died shortly after the experiment began, too soon to determine if the medication had any effect.

In fact, when Revici subsequently established himself in New York later that year, Freeman decided to join Revici. Dr. Freeman told me he spent, "a year to a year-and-a-half working with Revici" without pay.

Dr. Freeman said that he also went to New York to help run a family business. His father had recently died, so he decided to help out. Freeman told me he stopped working with Revici when he became satisfied that Revici's method hadn't been proven to work. It was also at this time that he realized that he had little interest in continuing to work in the family business. He informed his brother that he would no longer accept pay from the business.

Freeman and Revici also disagreed about how the research they were doing should be presented. The conflict may have played a significant role in Freeman's decision to leave. By the time Freeman joined Revici in New York he had already authored or co-authored 11 articles published in peer-review journals, including two in JAMA. His interest in having his findings published continued throughout his career with 102 published peer-review articles to his credit.

Freeman also found Revici's frequent leaping from one experiment to another more than a little disconcerting. A fountain of ideas, Revici would frustrate any number of his associates by constantly enhancing or even dropping an experiment in favor of a new one.

Despite Freeman's memory of his time in New York, it is quite possible that the reality of living in a Levittown community and his inability to produce publishable material while with Revici wore on him. He decided to return to mainstream medicine and academia, including a fruitful stint at the University Laboratory of Physical Chemistry at Harvard. Clearly, a scientist of Freeman's stature and abilities would not have connected himself to Revici if his track record was as the JAMA Council had stated.

In any event, it is not credible under any circumstances to believe that Dr. Freeman would have left a professorship at the prestigious University of Chicago Medical School to join Revici's independent research project without pay, if Revici's method had already failed with 52 patients. Dr. Freeman denies to this day that anything even resembling that figure ever took place. He said he had no idea where that figure came from, but indicated someone probably made it up.

Had there been 52 cases treated with the Revici Method, there would certainly have been a written record of them. There is none. Yet, in the absence of any record of any patients treated by Revici, JAMA's Council on Pharmacy and Chemistry decided to make a claim for which it had no substantiation.

There is no indication in the JAMA Council broadside as to how they arrived at their claim of 52 patients. No one had submitted a study to JAMA reporting on Revici's method. Neither had JAMA performed their own study or commissioned one. Thus, without supporting data, JAMA categorized Revici's work as one of the "Fables and Frauds" and grossly mischaracterized his method.

JAMA should have known that their article would significantly damage the reputation of a licensed physician. Because their assertions against Revici's method were so serious, it was incumbent upon them to be sure of their facts. At least their readership would have counted on them to do as much.

Ironically, the same JAMA Council article that condemned Revici was quite harsh in its appraisal of the harm done by various other so-called "Frauds" it had identified in its January 8th article. For example, of a Dr. John Emil Hett, the Council reported:

> If indeed, a cure for cancer had existed since 1931 as claimed by Dr. Hett, **then the responsibility of all the deaths from the disease since that time could be ascribed to his failure to make known his discovery to all other physicians.** (emphasis added)

Since it was JAMA, through its editors—not Revici—who has deterred his peers from learning of his cancer discoveries, one might inquire whether that same standard would apply to itself. As we have seen in the letters from some of the physicians who visited him in Mexico, Dr. Revici was more than accommodating to the physicians who were interested in his research. He did his best to inform them in a professional manner without promoting it to the public.

To this day, no correction of its egregious error has ever appeared within the covers of JAMA. Most doctors have not heard of Dr. Revici, and many of those who have heard of him think he is a quack, in no small part due to articles like the one that appeared in JAMA. It is interesting to note that others have quoted the 52-patient figure in subsequent articles, with the confidence that JAMA is their reliable source.

For example, Dr. Peter Byeff confidently testified against Revici in a court of law, saying he relied on the Journal as an authoritative source, and that Revici should have known therefore that his method was without merit. The American Cancer Society has also used the phantom figure as part of its reasoning for condemning Revici's method.

It wasn't long after the 1949 article appeared that the damage spread. The Brooklyn branch of the American Cancer Society quickly excerpted the 1949 JAMA article and sent it to Brooklyn area physicians. Sent as an advisory notice, it all but eliminated any chance that a patient in need of Revici's services would be referred to him by another Brooklyn physician. The reprinted excerpted article surely persuaded those doctors that Revici's method had been demonstrated to be worthless.

Moreover, the director of the Brooklyn branch of the American Cancer Society sent letters to various people who were known to be supporters and financial backers of Revici's new Institute of Applied Biology which was then located in Brooklyn. Because of JAMA's refusal to set the record straight, Revici's ability to gain acceptance by the mainstream medical and philanthropic communities was not helped.

Upon the advice of some of his influential supporters, Revici sued the Brooklyn Cancer Society for disseminating the material that defamed him and his associates. Dr. John Masterson, who was then the president of the Medical Society of the State of New York, became aware of the suit and suggested that two organizations fighting cancer shouldn't be fighting each other. He recommended that the two parties agree to arbitration, and thereby avoid the unseemly glare of publicity. The two parties accepted, and Masterson became the arbitrator.

The arbitration was decided in favor of Dr. Revici. In the process, Dr. Masterson was impressed enough with Revici's method that he soon became a board member of the IAB, joining such luminaries as the Hon. William B. Carswell, Associate Justice of the Appellate Division of the Supreme Court of New York, and the Honorable Edward Lazansky who was the Presiding Justice of the same court. (Sara Churchill, the daughter of former British Prime Minister Winston Churchill, also served on the board of the IAB at one time, as did Jacques Maritain, the noted French philosopher.)

After its 1949 article, the Journal of the American Medical Association remained silent about Revici and his method for a number of years. But JAMA would later demonstrate that it was not completely finished publishing negative articles regarding Dr. Revici. In 1965, JAMA published a highly unusual report of a study conducted by a group of physicians, led by Dr. David Lyall, who called themselves the

Clinical Appraisal Group (CAG). If the first two reports published in JAMA regarding Revici were merely errors committed by the editors of that magazine, the CAG report leaves little question as to where the general sentiments of the Journal lie.

But before they could fire their next salvo, the American Cancer Society stepped into the fray.

27

The American Cancer Society's Unproven Opinions

*Most patients would be satisfied with the anecdotal
experience of the rehardening of their vertebrae.
It might not fit the American Cancer Society's definition
of an objective benefit, but it is a healthy spine,
with solid bones in place of the jelly that was there before.*

THE AUTHOR

The vast majority of the American public trusts the American Cancer Society (ACS). Perhaps only the Red Cross and the Salvation Army are more highly regarded than this premier, private cancer organization. Its standing is so high that the Associated Press once ran a ten-part series of ACS press releases as if the releases were news, without indicating the ACS as the source of the information. The American Cancer Society also enjoys the support of a large number of volunteers nationwide. Perhaps, as a result of those factors, the non-profit American Cancer Society is perceived to have one of the finest reputations in the United States.

In recent years at least, the ACS has been near the forefront in the effort to get people to stop smoking, a major cause of cancer and other health problems, through its annual "Great American Smoke Out" campaign. Sponsorship of that event adds further credibility to their friendly image of doing their best to stop cancer. Their image of trustworthiness is even reflected in the obituaries of every newspaper where the bereaved will sometimes suggest that gifts be made to the ACS in lieu of sending flowers.

Yet there is another side to the ACS. That other side has played a significant role in limiting the average cancer specialist's access to the body of knowledge resulting from Dr. Revici's seminal research.

To understand the Society's conflicting attitudes, one must first consider who its founders were. The ACS took over in a friendly coup from the American Society for the Control of Cancer (ASCC) which also had some illustrious founders including the head of Standard Oil, John D. Rockefeller, who provided for the organization's initial financing in 1913. His grandson, Laurence Rockefeller, would hold the position of Honorary Chairman of Sloan-Kettering during the 1980's.

According to Ralph Moss, the founders of the ACS wanted to establish a more centralized control of the volunteer movement interested in finding a cure for cancer. By the early 1940's an ASCC branch group known as the Women's Field Army, a uniformed women's league of cancer volunteers, was being recognized as the predominant private non-profit organization in the fight against cancer. As Moss points out, while the ASCC had fewer than a thousand members, the grassroots Women's Field Army boasted a membership of over one million women.

In response to this burgeoning group of volunteer women, a group within the ASCC restructured the organization in 1944 and renamed itself the American Cancer Society. "One of the first things they did was to abolish the Women's Field Army and institute top-down control of all branches of the Society from its New York headquarters," Moss wrote in his benchmark book, *The Cancer Industry*. By centralizing the decision making, the founders of the ACS believed they would be better able to control the direction of cancer research and policy.

One ACS founder was Elmer Bobst, who started his career as a drug company representative. From that low-level beginning, he rose to become the president of the American wing of the giant pharmaceutical company, Hoffman-LaRoche. From there he became the president of yet another behemoth drug company, Warner-Lambert.

The relationship between former Hoffman-LaRoche president Bobst and the ACS has produced some interesting entanglements. According to Moss, the ACS became a 25% owner of the patent rights to the popular cancer drug 5-FU, which was manufactured by Hoffman-LaRoche. Color ads for 5-FU and other cancer drugs can be found on the back cover of a bimonthly ACS publication called *Ca: Cancer Journal for Clinicians*. After President Nixon declared an official war on cancer and signed the National Cancer Act on December 23, 1971, ACS co-founder and former pharmaceutical president, Bobst, was appointed to the National Cancer Advisory Board.

Another ACS co-founder was Albert Lasker, an advertising executive who coined the phrase, "Reach for a Lucky instead of a sweet," for the American Tobacco Company. Lasker's wife, Mary, was an extremely influential figure in Democratic politics with friendships that included Hubert Humphrey, Lyndon Johnson and other political heavyweights. According to Moss, Mrs. Lasker played a key role in the passage of the National Cancer Act.

Private and corporate donations now provide the ACS with several hundred million dollars annually. Meanwhile, the public is only dimly aware of the connections between the ACS and the drug industry. The ACS provides approximately $100 million dollars a year in research grants, much of it to fund drug studies.

According to Richard Carter, author of *The Gentle Legions* published in 1961, Dr. John Heller made the following statement in 1960:

> The Cancer Society and the National Cancer Institute work as partners. The Director of the Institute is a member of the board of directors of the Cancer Society, and the scientific advisory committees of both organizations interlock.

Dr. John Heller was first introduced in the chapter regarding Dr. Robert Fishbein. It was Heller who confessed to repeatedly seeing the positive effects of Dr. Revici's medicines in patients. Heller was also a director of the National Cancer Institute.

There is nothing illegal about a pharmaceutical president being at the center of the birth of the ACS. Nor is it illegal for its publications to be sponsored, in part, by advertisements for cancer drugs. Dual employment by the ACS and the National Cancer Institute is also apparently legal. But we must ask ourselves just what role we want an organization to play whose leadership might have a vested interest in which methods of cancer treatment are approved and which are not.

Of course, organizations can change, and the ACS is no exception. For a long time the Society had to be dragged kicking and screaming into recognizing the link between smoking and cancer, whereas now they sponsor the annual Great American Smoke Out. But there are other areas where the ACS allegiance seems to be the same as when the nonprofit Society was started in the mid 1940's.

Sometimes the ACS will even go to bat for drug firms. For example, Betsy Lehman was known as an aggressive consumer health reporter for the Boston Globe. She died at the age of 39 at Dana-Farber Hospital, one of the nation's premier cancer centers, after being given an overdose of chemotherapy on four consecutive days. Another patient, who was also overdosed at the same time, suffered severe heart damage.

Once the news of the overdoses finally broke several months later, damage control set in. On the television program, Good Morning America, a woman vice-president from the ACS fielded the host's questions. The ACS spokesperson told viewers that the way a person could protect themselves from being hurt accidentally from overdoses from chemotherapy was to, "Ask questions," without becoming a "pest."

One would assume that Ms Lehman was probably as well equipped as any patient to ask the right questions. Yet that was not enough to protect her from the dangers of the treatment she received. It was clear from the overall tone and demeanor of the ACS vice-president that her purpose was to quell people's fears regarding chemotherapy. It was unclear as to why the ACS found it necessary to interject itself into the issue in the first place.

But there is more to the ACS than its relationship with the pharmaceutical industry. As was envisioned by its founders, the ACS also has a major influence upon national medical policy and is heavily involved in establishing the way medicine is practiced in hospitals and in private physicians' offices across the U.S.

For example, in 1992 the ACS formally recommended that a test known as the Prostate Specific Antigen (PSA) be given routinely to all men over the age of fifty. Prior to the ACS recommendation, the test had the much more limited use of tracking prostate cancer patients to see if any relationship existed between increasing PSA scores and the progress of prostate cancer.

Physicians are divided about whether there is any benefit in treating most prostate cancer because of its slow growth. One deceased male out of every four over the age of 60 is found to have prostate cancer at the time of death—yet dies of other causes. Furthermore, studies have indicated that the treatment of prostate cancer has not necessarily increased patient longevity.

Because treatment often results in such problems as loss of bladder control, impotence, internal bleeding, and even diarrhea, many doctors often prefer an approach of "watchful waiting" when it comes to prostate cancer. By pushing for PSA tests for all men over 50, there is a real concern that doctors will feel pushed into taking action in many cases where inaction is the more healthful approach. It is believed by many physicians that, unless there are other symptoms, it is often best not to treat prostate cancer.

Once the ACS made its pronouncement, however, the PSA test for men over fifty practically became a requirement. University of Virginia Associate Professor of Medicine Andrew Wolfe, M.D., told the Washington Post, "Undiagnosed cancer is the number two or three cause of malpractice litigation, and when you have a major organization like that [ACS], it's not a law, but it can become a standard of care."

In fact, the medical profession relies heavily upon the editorial opinions of the ACS. The opinions expressed in such ACS journals such as *Ca: Cancer Journal for Clinicians* can become the minimum standard of practice for those physicians who are wishing to avoid unnecessary lawsuits.

As the Washington Post health writer, Rick Weiss, pointed out, the ACS decision to support routine PSA testing came after companies with a direct financial interest in the testing and treatment of prostate cancer paid for a four-day meeting at an exclusive resort hotel for ACS officials. Although opinions regarding the benefit of administering routine PSA testing based upon age is still quite divided, the published recommendation by a committee of the ACS prevails as a practical matter.

The official opinions of the American Cancer Society might appear to be somewhat innocuous. One could argue that although support for the PSA test might mean significantly increased costs for medical care with little or no demonstrably proven benefits, it does not hurt to err on the side of caution. But the larger question concerns whether a private organization—whose ties to private industries might influence its decisions—should have so much say in determining medical standards.

The ACS's heavy influence over medical procedures is only one area where the ACS affects medical policy. In addition to recommending specific tests, the ACS also discredits treatment methods it does not support. In Revici's case, the ACS warned practicing physicians and their patients to avoid the Revici Method by declaring that it was an "Unproven Method."

The ACS committee responsible for the "Unproven Methods" articles is "the committee on quackery" according to the courtroom testimony of Victor Herbert, M.D., a legally-trained physician who has been a member of that committee. In fact, Dr. Herbert made that announcement in his role as an expert witness against Revici in a lawsuit. Herbert's statement leaves little doubt as to the purpose of the ACS's "Unproven Methods" articles, at least as it applied to Dr. Revici.

The first "Unproven Methods" article regarding Dr. Revici appeared in the March/April issue of 1961 in the ACS medical journal, *Ca: Cancer Journal for Clinicians*. The two-page article was entitled, "Unproven Methods of Cancer Treatment." After superficially describing Revici's theory in a single paragraph and devoting half of the short article to a skeletal biography of Revici's life and career, the two-page statement ended with the following conclusion regarding his method of treatment:

After careful study of the literature and other information available to it, the American Cancer Society has found no acceptable evidence that treatment with the Revici Cancer Control results in any objective benefit in the treatment of cancer in human beings.

The ACS tacitly admitted that it had no scientific evidence upon which to base its opinion by complaining, "Since 1944 repeated attempts have been made by many individuals and groups to set up studies.... In every case it has been impossible to reach [an] agreement...."

The article failed to mention that the proponents of those studies wanted to test individual medicines without applying the dualistic principles that must be used to ensure their effectiveness. In other words, studies were proposed that would prescribe a single medication for a patient without regard for the patient's acid/alkaline imbalance. The proposed studies were, literally speaking, fatally flawed in their design, so Revici refused to agree to a test under those circumstances.

The article also criticized Revici for utilizing 17 different substances in his attack against cancer and said "no agent or agents to control cancer of *either type* has been reported as an agent of choice for long," (emphasis added) and faulted him for wanting all 17 tested by a "group which was trying to reach an agreement with the Institute...."

The ACS opinion seemed to be that Revici should have found a single agent "of choice." That opinion indicated their own bias for a set regimen approach of applying a single agent for a preset amount of time. The criticism was apparently an unwitting admission by the ACS that they had no understanding of how to apply Revici's method, nor did they understand the dualistic and hierarchic organizational underpinnings of the method.

The ACS criticism failed to take into account one of the fundamental differences between Revici's approach to cancer therapy and the one used by others. Standard chemotherapy protocols are fairly rigid in their application in that patients are given a preset amount of one or more cancer drugs for a fixed number of treatments.

As Revici's term "biologically guided" would indicate, his protocol varies from patient to patient and from day to day. Revici's method uses the biological feedback of the patient to determine the course of each patient's indivualized treatment.

Dr. Revici has emphasized repeatedly the importance of tailoring each treatment based on frequent test results, which may be conducted *several times a day*. Revici has made it abundantly clear in lectures, articles and in his book that he doesn't rely on a single medication, but on a method of treatment.

The unsigned ACS article was sent to 120,000 cancer specialists and treatment centers and, "to the 60 Divisions of the American Cancer Society for their information." Although it is not mentioned in the article, there is evidence that the American Cancer Society had at its disposal an advance copy of Revici's book.

For example, the brief article referred to Revici's treatment as "biologically guided chemotherapy," a term he first introduced in his book. Dr. Revici also has said that the ACS was sent an advance copy prior to the article's appearance.

But arguing the merits of Revici's book and method might miss the larger point. Revici had no forum to adequately respond to the ACS. Their article was sent to a much larger audience of cancer specialists than he had access to. Of course, Revici's text was written with that same medical audience in mind.

The ACS, with its huge budget, had spent neither time nor money to scientifically confirm or refute his work. Yet, once the targeted audience of oncologists had been blanketed, there was little he could do. Revici might have had a better understanding of the science than the ACS, but the field of battle wasn't a scientific one. It was a battle of public relations, which the ACS won easily.

Just like the PSA test mentioned earlier, the opinion of the ACS regarding Revici's method had the effect of influencing the nation's cancer practitioners to heed its opinion. The unspoken message was clear: A practitioner better think twice before considering the Revici method for his own patients. Similarly, hospitals would be reluctant to allow the practice of Revici's method at their institutions.

It is worth noting the significance of the anonymous authorship of the ACS article. Exactly who was behind the ACS article remains unknown except at the American Cancer Society headquarters. The article was prepared by the anonymous members of the Medical Affairs Subcommittee on Questionable Methods of Cancer Management, previously known as the Committee on Unproven Methods.

The ACS does not list the names of those members anywhere in its publications. When asked, the ACS refused to release the names of the authors of the article. I requested the names of the author[s] of the articles regarding Dr. Revici, but a spokesperson at the national office in Atlanta informed me that the policy of the ACS was that the names would not be released without the permission of the individual committee members.

The anonymous article on Revici had the very real effect of moving the discussion of the efficacy of his method from the realm of science into a college fraternity blackball. Without performing a single scientific test of their own, or relying on any scientific testing by anyone else, the ACS declaration had the effect of categorizing Revici as a quack. As a result of that declaration, the ACS greatly reduced any chance that Revici's book would be seriously considered by the nation's cancer practitioners.

A less influential organization also considered his book. The board of trustees of an international organization known as "The Society for the Promotion of International Scientific Relations" included 14 members who had either already earned the Nobel prize in science or who would subsequently win it. This board was much more impressed with Dr. Revici's book. The board awarded Dr. Revici its annual medal six months after the ACS found his work wanting.

One other scientist with an even tinier voice added his assessment. After reading the book, a Revici associate came to him and told him that he counted 113 new discoveries that were included in it.

Whatever spin one might place on the motivations of the ACS, the fact is that Revici's book went largely unread. Fewer than 500 total copies were sold either domestically or internationally. Still, the questions arise, "What if Revici's text had been seen by the nation's oncologists? What would those doctors have seen?"

They would have seen photographic copies of Mrs. E.H.'s spinal x-rays beginning on page 487. The x-ray shows where E.H.'s cancer had chewed on and turned into jelly a large portion of three of the vertebrae in the middle of her back. In addition, part of her left collar bone had been assaulted, as well as two of her ribs, her pelvis and her thigh bones. Two pages later those doctors would have then seen x-ray evidence of the same patient's regenerated backbone—a whole and complete, perfectly shaped spine with a rehardening of the bones *in just four months time*. Continuing on in the book, the doctors would have seen considerable bone repair to E. H.'s pelvis, ribs, collar and thigh bones.

Had those physicians continued, they would have read that E.H., who had been paralyzed by her disease and in great pain, had become completely pain-free and able to walk without a brace or cane. From their own experience of treating cancer patients, any cancer doctors reading Revici's book in 1961 would have realized that E.H.'s spectacular recovery was unparalleled in their own practices.

Flipping the pages a little further, they would have seen the skull x-ray of another patient which contained numerous holes caused by the spread of cancer. Turning the page, the doctors would have seen the same skull. Only this time the holes were gone because her skull had healed and her tumor was gone. These doctors would have known from their medical training that conventional medicine had no drug at that time that could produce similar results. Possibly their curiosity would have been piqued to know how Revici's treatments could perform in ways that modern medicines could not.

Had those doctors continued to turn the pages, they would have seen more x-rays of Revici's patients whose ribs, hips, arms and legs came back to life and grew fresh, healthy bones. With each case, some of those doctors would have had to ask themselves if those kinds of remarkable results were possible with common medical treatments. Each time their answer would have been a resounding, "No!" In many cases, the best those doctors could hope for would be to relieve some of the patient's pain before he or she died—and there was even no guarantee of that.

The likelihood of conventional practitioners seeing in their own practices the widespread bone regeneration—which Revici frequently achieved—was next to none, if not impossible. But it was not just healed bones the doctors would have learned about. The doctors would have also noticed that Revici's patients did not have to deal with the widespread side effects of chemotherapy, surgery and radiation, such as prolonged diarrhea, world-class nausea, severe upper respiratory conditions, radiation-induced burns and broken bones, loss of bladder control, loss of appetite, painful mouth sores, impotence, ruptured blood vessels, paralysis, amputations, and others too numerous to mention.

They would have also learned that Revici's patients typically became pain-free without narcotics or other pain killers as their bodies healed. The doctors would have known from their own practices that they had no medicine that could accomplish this dual effect. To the contrary, they would have been left to compare their own patients who were doubled-over in pain with nausea, bleeding gums, and unable to eat.

If the American Cancer Society was unwilling to accept x-ray evidence of complete, simultaneous bone regeneration at several sites as "acceptable evidence" of an "objective benefit," just what were they looking for that would have convinced them? Many patients would be satisfied with the anecdotal experience of the rehardening of their vertebrae. It might not fit the American Cancer Society's definition of an "objective benefit," but it is a healthy spine with solid bones in place of the jelly that was there before. If such a feat of multiple bone reformation were accomplished by using the latest industry-backed chemotherapy or radiation treatment, the event would certainly be heralded on the network news and in every newspaper and magazine as a medical triumph of historic proportions.

The purpose of this book is not to find and expose the motivations of those who have stood in the way of Revici's method. Yet, in researching and writing this book, I have been besieged by that question from others. It seems that people want to know who the villains are. Furthermore, they just can't believe a cure for cancer would be suppressed.

I am providing the historical data in the hope that the reader can understand how it is possible that Revici's discoveries have been squelched. But I am more interested in raising these discoveries up for the public to see, than I am in looking for the fingerprints of the guilty. It is obvious that certain people have impeded Revici—the evidence that his method is superior to mainstream medicine is shockingly clear—but focusing on finger-pointing wastes time that could be spent promoting progress.

Some would say there is too much money involved to let an independent medical researcher come up with a superior treatment for cancer. Whether that is true or not is for the reader to decide. For most people it is indeed difficult to imagine that an organization like the ACS, with its large base of volunteer support, would cruelly let people suffer and die even if a great deal of money were involved.

The idea that money controls the American Cancer Society has a problem in that it smears a legion of dedicated, caring people who are as prone to the same illnesses as the rest of us. In the case of the American Cancer Society's criticisms of Revici's method, it was not the whole ACS community of workers and supporters that tarred his name and method without the benefit of scientific support. It was a few people taking advantage of the cover of secrecy.

Who knows, it is even possible that those who were responsible actually believed that they were protecting Americans from some potential danger. Those few people, whether acting on good faith or bad, had the power to determine whether or not Revici's method would receive a fair reading by the medical community.

In 1971, the ACS reprinted an updated version of the article it printed in 1961. The 1971 article mentioned a study conducted by a group that called itself the CAG which will be discussed in the next chapter at length. In reference to the CAG study the ACS wrote, "A detailed criticism of this report has been issued by Dr. Revici."

Considering the impact of the "Unproven Methods" articles, it would be incumbent upon the ACS to be at least somewhat familiar with Revici's critique before going forward with its articles. The reader will discover in the next chapter that their knowledge of the Revici critique also points to their culpability in their effort to dismiss Revici's work. As the reader shall see, anyone familiar with Revici's critique of the CAG would be hard pressed to honestly use the CAG report as a basis for an argument against Revici's method.

Another 400,000 practitioners were notified of Revici's method in 1989 by the American Cancer Society through yet another, longer "Unproven Methods" article regarding Revici's work.*

The 1989 ACS attack stated bluntly, "[T]he American Cancer Society strongly urges individuals with cancer not to seek treatment with the Revici Method." The phantom 52 patients also reappeared with an accompanying JAMA footnote. [See Chapter 26.]

The "Mexican treatment" letter [Discussed in Chapter 25] was also rehashed. The article also falsely stated, "[Trafalgar] Hospital was suspended from the Medicaid program for fraud." As its source the ACS supplied a footnote referring to the New York Daily News, an unusual source for a scientific journal. Yet the Daily News made no mention of fraud charges in its article. Thus, the ACS misquoted a tabloid newspaper as its source for character assassination of Dr. Revici's reputation.

Although the local Medicaid office did question certain payments made to Trafalgar Hospital regarding the drug treatment program referred to in Chapter 9, the final disposition of the matter ended with Medicaid making further payments to the hospital. At no time were charges of fraud filed against the hospital or any of its employees, including Dr. Revici.

The American Cancer Society also erroneously claimed that Revici treated cancer with soft boiled eggs and coffee. The accusation further demonstrated their lack of familiarity with Revici's method.

Revici had learned through his research that both soft boiled eggs and coffee are concentrated anabolic foods. As discussed previously, one of Revici's earliest findings was that patients with anabolic pain worsened when treated with an anabolic substance but improved when treated with a catabolic substance.

---

* The 1989 article quotes from the CAG critique by Revici, an additional piece of evidence that the ACS authors had access to the critique. Revici's critique so thoroughly discredits the CAG report that its use by the ACS against Revici defies all logic, had their intent been scientific in nature.

Conversely, patients with catabolic pain had a lessening of their pain when treated with an anabolic substance, but had a worsening of their pain if treated with a catabolic substance.

Revici used that knowledge as a means of helping to monitor patients—who were already under care and who had called from home —to help determine if they were exhibiting either an anabolic or catabolic pain pattern at that moment. On those occasions Revici would advise a patient to eat an egg and to drink some coffee. He would also instruct them to call him back to let him know if the prescribed meal caused the patient to feel better or worse. For Revici the coffee and eggs were prescribed for the sole purpose of making an up-to-the-moment determination of the patient's anabolic/catabolic condition.

Revici knew that his suggested diet would make an anabolic pain pattern temporarily feel worse while making a catabolic one temporarily feel better. With that information he could advise the patient which medicine to take, if any, as well as to determine if the patient might need to come in to see him again. In 74 years of medical practice, Revici has never used soft boiled eggs and coffee to *treat* cancer, but only as a quick way to monitor and identify the patient's overall condition, and to help the patient avoid an unnecessary trip to the office.

Despite the continued wild inaccuracies spread about him, Revici did not attempt to fight back. It is supremely ironic, in an era where the scientific method has become the centerpiece of medicine, that a true scientist can be ostracized and vilified by the ACS without its having to rely on accurate scientific data. Yet, the facts speak for themselves. In all of its pronouncements, the only scientific article relied upon by the ACS to discredit Revici's method was the CAG report— a report that it should have known to be worthless.

Whether or not a quest for either money or scientific truths are factors in keeping Revici's methods from the medical community and the public, there is another factor that goes to the heart of Revici's difficulties with JAMA and the ACS.

In the nineteenth century, when a Hungarian doctor named Ignaz Semmelweis pleaded with other doctors to wash and disinfect their hands between performing autopsies and delivering babies, he ran into a type of resistance of the most unexpected kind. At that time, part of a doctor's status came from wiping his bloody hands on the lapels of his white lab coat. Although it sounds bizarre by today's standards, a large amount of dried blood on a doctor's lab coat conferred prestige upon him. Defending their most visible sign of status, Semmelweis's blood-encrusted superiors refused to accept his findings. After bumping heads with the recalcitrant medical establishment, Dr. Semmelweis became ostracized in his own country.

The ignorance and stubbornness of the times resulted in a continual epidemic for pregnant women who often died of childbirth fever after being infected by the dirty hands of their doctors. After more than a decade of trying unsuccessfully to convince his profession of the need for antiseptic practices and distraught by the unnecessary deaths of pregnant women, Semmelweis went mad and died in an insane asylum. Only much later did Pasteur prove Semmelweis's theory to be correct.

Much like Semmelweis's detractors, the well-thought-of American Cancer Society has spoken, and its well-circulated arguments have carried the day. Meanwhile, today's cancer patients are a bit like the defenseless women of Dr. Semmelweis's era.

Four years after the first of the ACS's critiques of Revici's method appeared, a prominent medical professor would spearhead the CAG report against Revici's method in a peer-review article that would be published by JAMA. The next chapter will reveal for the first time publicly how this small group of physicians was able to provide the so-called scientific evidence that Revici's method was worthless.

28

Lyall and the Truth

"[H]e said to my husband and me, 'You know this isn't going to work. In fact I've even been offered $10,000 to see this fail.... I never did find out who offered it... but I bet he accepted it."

TESTIMONY BY ETHEL PRATT DURING AN OFFICE OF
PROFESSIONAL MEDICAL CONDUCT HEARING REGARDING
A CONVERSATION WITH JON GREGG, DR. LYALL'S MESSENGER

"It was a disgrace."

CUSHMAN HAAGENSEN, M.D.,
REFERRING TO THE CAG STUDY

On October 18, 1965, an important medical event took place. On that day the results of a scientific study were published in the Journal of the American Medical Association regarding Dr. Revici's method. The study was signed by lead author, David Lyall, M.D., and several other physicians. Above the article's headline was a two word summary: "Negative Results." The report stated unequivocally that the Revici method was completely ineffective in helping any of the 33 patients included in the report.

The study was critically important because it was supposed to be the first published scientific look at the Revici Method. It also meant that it was no longer necessary to rely on anecdotal accounts to determine its effectiveness. Anyone who was interested in knowing the value of Revici's method could be directed to the study published in JAMA. The interested reader would see that once it was subjected to a legitimate scientific trial, the Revici Method was proved worthless.

There was one rather large problem with Lyall's article, however—the report was significantly at odds with the actual results experienced by the patients, so JAMA's readership was greatly misled. Moreover, a large number of medical records pointed to a stunning breach of medical ethics.

Nine physicians supposedly co-authored the JAMA article. Yet, one of those authors called the entire study "a disgrace." Another was privately so impressed with Revici's method he had written a favorable letter about it to the President of the United States. A third, later testifying in court that he never saw any slides and photos, said he would have changed his opinion if he had seen them. The pathologist of the study apparently rarely, if ever, saw a microscopic slide, x-ray, photo or autopsy report. Yet another physician admitted in court that the lead researcher and sole author of the CAG report never showed any medical evidence of any patient's progress to any of the other co-authors.

The chief architect of the Clinical Appraisal Group (CAG)—who would refer to his study as a model for other doctors to follow in the future—was New York University Professor of Medicine, David Lyall, M.D. Stephen Schwartz, M.D., also from NYU, acted as his right-hand man.

Prior to the American Cancer Society's "Unproven Methods" article in 1961, there may have been little need for the CAG study at all. Revici's 1961 text might have opened up all sorts of inquiries from interested members of his profession. The book was teeming with scientific leads. As Morris A. Mann, M.D., has written:

> A number of my colleagues, who are like myself involved in molecular design, have had access to his work, and all have indicated that Dr. Revici is a major contributor to our understanding of structure/function relationships in pharmacology.

After widespread readership of Revici's book within the medical community, it is also likely that Dr. Welt's series of studies [See Chapter 24] would have been one among many to introduce Dr. Revici's theories and applications to other interested scientists and physicians.

Revici's institute had enjoyed for a time the enthusiastic support of a small number of well-heeled backers. On at least three occasions in the 1950's the New York Times had reported on highly successful fund-raising efforts that were held to support Revici's research. With the combined support of newly-interested medical people and researchers, along with private and institutional donors, the progressive spread of Revici's theories and practices would have undoubtedly continued to this day.

However, the ACS article did appear, and as a result the expected professional boost from his book failed to materialize. Over time it became increasingly difficult for Revici to maintain his small cadre of support, especially when his backers had hoped Revici's method would soon become widely accepted and not reviled, as it had become in professional medical circles.

The damage caused by the earlier JAMA articles and the American Cancer Society particularly affected the IAB's ability to attract new donors. Adding new donors was important because Revici's treatments were often not covered by insurance, and the institute would not turn anyone away due to an inability to pay for treatment, a policy Revici insisted on.

But finding donors was not always easy. According to Marcus Cohen, the well known radio announcer, Walter Winchell, considered supporting Revici. When Winchell asked someone whom he trusted in the medical field about Revici, Winchell's advisor steered him away and suggested that he contribute to the American Cancer Society instead.

Mrs. Ethel Pratt reported a similar type of situation within her own social circles. Her husband's grandfather, Charles Pratt, had been a member of the Standard Oil Trust. Her husband, Sherman Pratt, became a philanthropist for a number of causes. Besides being an active member of the IAB Board and volunteering her time four mornings a week, Mrs. Pratt also provided the board with generous financial support. In fact, her total financial contribution to the IAB over the years was well into the hundreds of thousands of dollars and might have reached as high as seven figures. In my visit to her home, Mrs. Pratt recalled the difficulty she had in interesting any of her friends from the country club in becoming fellow supporters, "They wanted to go with the crowd. Memorial [Sloan-Kettering] was where everyone wanted to associate."

As a result of the deteriorating financial situation and the repeated bad medical press, it became increasingly important that Revici demonstrate the effectiveness of his compounds through an objective study.

In 1962, Revici convinced the IAB board and its contributors to fund a study that would prove the value of his method. Because of the ongoing success he had achieved with hundreds of patients, Revici was confident that a thorough study would prove the superiority of his method and garner needed support for the Institute. Such an event would place Revici's work forever on the scientific map. From that initiative, a two-year study was set up to test its efficacy. The study, which would become known as the CAG report, was conducted from January of 1963 to December of 1964. It was understood by all concerned that the study, if successful, would serve to demonstrate a method that could be reproduced by other cancer specialists.

Dr. Revici would treat the patients at Trafalgar Hospital and have the progress and results examined by a team of five physicians led by Dr. David Lyall. According to the written protocol agreed to by Revici and Lyall, any changes made in the protocol would have to be agreed to in writing by both Dr. Revici and by the group.

Yet, the number of physicians associated with the CAG ballooned to nine members despite Dr. Revici's opposition. Although Revici never gave his permission to Dr. Lyall to add four more doctors, the additional names would appear on the final report published in JAMA.

The agreement stipulated that the sole criterion for determining the success of the trial would be made by measuring any tumor shrinkage. Cancer experts know that tumor shrinkage is the most difficult of all criteria to achieve. Weight gain, elimination of pain, and increase of life expectancy were not to be considered by the CAG. Still, Revici readily agreed to tumor shrinkage as the sole criteria for the study because he had already done that with hundreds of other patients.

To understand how Lyall was able to control the reported results, it is first necessary to take a look at some of the conditions under which the study was conducted.

The first important circumstance that allowed duplicity to occur came about because, with one exception, only Dr. Lyall and Dr. Schwartz saw any of the patients. Dr. Herter saw one patient on two occasions at Delafield Hospital. The other six co-author/physicians never examined or saw a single patient during the entire length of the two-year study. As it turned out, the absentee stewardship by most of the co-authors would play heavily into Lyall's ability to control the reported progress of the patients.

The meeting place for the discussion of the patients' progress was also unusual. One would expect scientists, whose names were to appear on a peer-review article, to conduct their research in a lab, a hospital or an examining room. This was not the case.

According to later court testimony from Dr. Frederic Herter and Dr. Jane Wright, Lyall would report whatever findings he had to the other doctors at bimonthly dinner meetings at the Overseas Press Club in Manhattan. In all, twelve dinners were held. Dr. Revici was not permitted to attend any of these meetings.

Copies of the dinner checks for three of those meetings have been recovered. According to the restaurant bill from the first meeting, held on January 9, 1963, the four attending doctors ordered twenty-seven shots of liquor and a bottle of wine, or an average of eight alcoholic drinks per attending physician.

By July of 1963, the CAG group grew to nine dinner attendees. At that meeting, twenty-six shots of liquor and two bottles of wine were ordered, according to the restaurant tab—the equivalent of three or more drinks for each CAG co-author. Of course some of the attendees might have abstained from drinking alcohol, making the average for those who did drink higher still.

A third meeting, held in February of 1964, indicates twenty shots and two bottles of wine for a party of six, or an average of five alcoholic drinks per scientist present.

The dinner parties were the only meetings that were held to discuss patient progress, according to court testimony by two of the co-authors. As can be seen by the fluctuating attendance at the dinner meetings, input from all the doctors was apparently not necessary.

According to a report prepared by Dr. Revici in late 1965, nearly 25% of the sum for the twelve dinner bills charged by the CAG group to Trafalgar Hospital was for alcohol. When the three available dinner bills are examined, the picture becomes more telling. When extraneous expenditures like cigars, flowers and room charges are removed, the alcohol portion of the bills is nearly 40%, not an inconsiderable portion of the total bill when one realizes that single shots at the Overseas Press Club were selling for eighty-five and ninety-five cents a drink at that time.

According to testimony given in a court proceeding, Dr. Lyall would give an oral report to the other doctors. The attending dinner guest/researchers were never provided with any visual medical evidence of microscopic slides, x-rays, photographs or any other documentation. With the exception of Dr. Schwartz, the other doctors would have no input because they had not seen any of the patients. Court testimony by Dr. Herter and Dr. Wright indicates that the other doctors accepted the reports of Dr. Lyall at face value.

At the second dinner meeting, Dr. Cushman Haagensen of Columbia University College of Physicians and Surgeons made it clear he did not want to have his name associated with the study, although Dr. Lyall tried to convince him otherwise. While Haagensen firmly believed Revici's method was totally ineffective, he apparently recognized the unprofessional circumstances of the study and wanted no part of it. Haagensen was so adamant in his desire to have his name disassociated with the study that his refusal was inserted into the protocol: "Dr. Haagensen indicated his firm decision not to appear as a member of the CAG... [H]e would not wish to associate himself with any report made by the Group... "

That insertion with the protocol is consistent with the minutes of the second meeting of the CAG which stated, "For a number of reasons, Dr. Haagensen felt he did not wish his name to appear as a member of the group, and that further he would not wish to associate himself with any reports made by this group."

One can speculate as to why Haagensen would feel the need to make his desires a part of the protocol after clearly stating them at a CAG meeting. Is it possible that Haagensen suspected Lyall would put his name on the study without his permission?

In fact, that is exactly what Lyall did. Despite Haagensen's refusal to be associated with the report, his name, along with the eight others, appeared atop the CAG article criticizing the Revici Method. Years later, when he was asked about the report by Dr. Alice Ladas, whose husband was under Revici's care, Dr. Haagensen replied, "It was a disgrace," and added that his name should never have appeared as a co-author of the article.

At least two other doctors, whose names were on the report, disagreed with its contents. Dr. John Galbraith, another influential physician who was a former president of the Nassau County Medical Society, also appeared as a signer to the CAG study. Dr. Galbraith had known of the Revici Method since at least 1951 and had spoken on its behalf at a fund-raising dinner at that time, according to a New York Times article.

In June of 1963, Galbraith sent a hand-written note to Dr. Revici regarding three patients who were not part of the study and who were not treated with the Revici Method. The first patient was Galbraith's own wife, who died of cancer. In the letter Galbraith told Revici her death was the result of her not taking the medicine Revici had prescribed. Galbraith then went on to say he believed she would have gotten well if she would have only taken her medicine.

In the same letter, Galbraith referred to two other patients he was privately treating using the Revici Method who were gradually improving as a result.

Galbraith wrote at least two other letters in support of Revici as well. In 1959, he learned that the U.S. Secretary of State, John Foster

Dulles, had cancer. Galbraith took it upon himself to write President Eisenhower and implored the President to have Dulles get in contact with Mrs. Pratt, who was on the board of the IAB at that time. Galbraith told Eisenhower, "I've seen dramatic changes in the course of cancer in two patients," with Revici's method. He added that he was treating "several of my patient.... by this method." The tone of the letter to the president clearly indicated that Galbraith's opinion was the opposite of that contained in the CAG report.

Two weeks later Galbraith addressed a letter to a physician affiliated with Columbia-Presbyterian. The letter indicated that the two had been at a meeting where some of Revici's patients were the topic of discussion. It is evident from the letter that the other doctor had expressed the opinion that the patients discussed at the previous meeting might have improved for reasons other than Revici's treatment. Galbraith defended the effectiveness of Revici's method in the letter, arguing that the patients' improvements were directly correlated to the time of Revici's treatment.

The dates of the various letters suggest Galbraith had used some of Revici's compounds for a period of at least five years. A letter written by Ethel Pratt, who had been a long-time patient of Galbraith, indicates that his use of Revici's methods on his own patients went on for at least nine years. Each Galbraith letter reported positive results due to Revici's compounds. It is rather unlikely that the politically aware Galbraith would have continued to use Revici's controversial method for that length of time if he had not found it to be superior to other methods that were available.

Galbraith was not immune to the social and political pressures of associating with Revici, however. For example, during the period when Dr. Galbraith's wife was seen by Revici at Trafalgar Hospital, she was treated under an assumed name, according to patient, Robert Fishbein, M.D. In addition, Dr. Galbraith confided to Ethel Pratt that he allowed his name to be added to the CAG report because he, "couldn't go against all the others."

The lack of documentation provided to the co-authors played a critical part in some of the physicians' willingness to add their names to the report. CAG co-author Frederic Herter, M.D., later testified before the New York State Office of Professional Medical Conduct in 1984 at a license revocation hearing regarding Dr. Revici. He told the panel that if he had seen the photographs and biopsies of the CAG patients presented to him at the hearings, he would have changed his verdict and not signed the report.

A fourth signer, Dr. Jane Wright, corroborated Herter's testimony by admitting, while testifying as a witness in a medical malpractice suit, that neither she nor the other doctors were shown any photos or other lab results at the dinner gatherings or at any other time.

Other than the possible inebriation of CAG members and the lack of information provided by Lyall, little is known about the conduct and demeanor of any of the dinner meeting attendees. The reason for the lack of knowledge regarding the meetings is that Lyall refused to provide the minutes of those meetings to Revici, to the Trafalgar Board, or to the IAB. In point of fact, it is unknown if any minutes were actually taken at any of the meetings except for the meeting where Haagensen made a point of being excluded from the group's membership. A great deal more is known about Dr. Lyall's behavior at Trafalgar Hospital.

One of the patients who was just beginning treatment at Trafalgar at that time was Robert Fishbein, M.D., the brain tumor patient whose story was told earlier (Chapter 12). In fact, because of his rapid recovery, Fishbein soon became a regular volunteer at Trafalgar. He would become a second set of eyes as to the activities of Dr. Lyall and Dr. Schwartz. At the end of the two years, he was so taken aback by Lyall's behavior that he decided to write his own report on the CAG. In the introduction to that report, Fishbein wrote in his typically understated manner:

> Because what was suspected as early as January 1964 and became apparent by November 1964, that the report of this Group would conclude that Dr. Revici's therapy had no value in the treatment of cancer, it seemed that my observation during this period should be presented in order to add clarity to the situation.

Fishbein's 24-page report contains numerous instances of activities that might call into question Lyall's intentions. In it Fishbein recounted the activities of Dr. Lyall regarding eighteen different patients.

For his part, Dr. Revici wrote several responses to Lyall's reports as well. Two of Revici's responses to Lyall's report are backed up by photos, biopsy reports, and/or autopsy reports to support each of his claims. In contrast, Dr. Lyall *never released any documented evidence* in support of the CAG report.

Together, the Fishbein and Revici reports provide two physicians' accounts of the attitude and practices of Dr. Lyall during the CAG study.

Revici's first response was an answer to Lyall's unpublished preliminary report. Lyall refused to tell Revici to whom he had sent his preliminary report, a violation of the original agreement. More importantly, Lyall refused to allow Revici to see either his notes or the numerous photos demonstrating patient progress that Revici had lent him. Despite Revici's repeated requests, Lyall never returned the photographic evidence he had in his possession from any of the cases.

Lyall's preliminary report, which was sent to an unknown number of medical reviewers, contained several patients who were never part of the CAG study, including one critically ill patient located at another hospital who died without ever receiving any treatment from Revici.

In one copy of a nineteen-page summary report written by Revici which was hand-dated "11/30/65," he briefly discussed the flaws in Lyall's actions during the two-year study, as well as the errors in Lyall's final report which had been published six weeks earlier in JAMA. This author made a conservative count of Lyall's alleged unethical actions mentioned in Revici's report. In the case of some of the questionable activities mentioned in Revici's summary, it is impossible to tell how many times Lyall repeated each particular activity.

For example, there is no indication of how many photos Lyall refused to turn over to Revici, although there were many. Although any one set of the photos might clearly indicate Lyall's alleged duplicity, this author counted Lyall's refusal to turn over all the sets of photos as only one act. Using that method I counted exactly 100 acts which, if true, would be possible grounds for professional disciplinary action—if not criminal charges.

Some of Revici's accusations, many of which were supported by third-party documented evidence, indicate that Lyall's reportage was at complete variance with the evidence. In the case of one patient, who will be discussed more fully later on in this chapter, Lyall noted, "[a] gradual increase in size of [the] tumor during course of therapy." Yet a series of dated photographic evidence this author has seen clearly showed an externally visible tumor which protruded from the patient's rectum and which dramatically disappeared over two-months' time. The disappearance of the tumor is mentioned nowhere in the final CAG report, although a change in tumor size was the only yardstick for measuring the success of the treatment method.

Dr. Revici prepared another rebuttal that ran over 100 pages, including copies of autopsy reports, photographic evidence, biopsy reports, etc. This report was a devastating rebuttal both to Lyall's preliminary and published reports.

We also learn from Revici's rebuttals that once he began to suspect Lyall's motives, he began to take his own photos of patients which were dated and signed on the back by Dr. Schwartz, one of the CAG co-authors. It is for that reason alone that any photos were available to Revici to help substantiate his arguments.

Some of the many flaws, alleged breeches of ethics, and the misinterpretations made by Lyall are worthy of analysis patient-by-patient. Only in that way will the reader be able to see the extent to which the published report could have misinformed JAMA's readership.

For example, Fishbein relates that in at least two different cases Dr. Lyall tried to convince patients who were responding to Revici's treatment to abandon it, nonetheless. One such case was James Alden* who had a Stage III cancer of both vocal chords. The tumors had punched a hole between his windpipe and his esophagus, and had spread to his skin. He had received no treatment prior to coming to Revici.

His lack of prior medical treatment made his case an important one for the study, because it could not be claimed later on that he had benefited from prior treatment. He began treatment with Revici and was

___

* The patient names in this chapter are pseudonyms.

presented to Lyall and Schwartz during their next visit. According to Fishbein's report:

> They advised the patient that he had neglected to get proper orthodox treatment. Mr. [Alden] became perplexed. Subsequent sessions with Drs. Schwartz and Lyall for the purpose of appraising the treatment resulted in further advice to Mr. [Alden] that he should have his tumor surgically removed at the earliest possible time. The anxiety was apparent in this individual who was confronted with a situation in violation of medical ethics.

Alden remained under treatment for six months before he dropped out of the study. He returned to Trafalgar later where he died of pneumonia. The autopsy showed that the only cancer remaining at the time of his death was a two-and-a-half-inch patch of cancerous skin. No tumor was found in either of his vocal chords or in any other organ, and the hole in his wind pipe, "was no longer visible," according to Revici. According to the study's protocol, the disappearance of the tumor from both sides of Alden's throat should have been recorded as a treatment success.

A woman who had a Stage II tumor of the tongue received similar advice from Lyall and Schwartz. Like Alden she also had no treatment prior to coming under Revici's care, except for a biopsy to confirm her diagnosis. According to Dr. Fishbein:

> Individually and together, Drs. Lyall and Schwartz advised the patient other forms of therapy were more desirable. On numerous occasions she was told by them that radiation or surgical intervention should be done at the earliest possible time.

After persistent persuasion by the two doctors, she left the study and was lost to follow up.

On January 21, 1964, 46-year-old Rebecca Turner was diagnosed by Dr. Cushman Haagensen as having bilateral breast cancer. Haagensen informed her that the tumors were inoperable, but that she should have her ovaries removed to prevent the spread of the tumor to those organs. The procedure was performed two weeks later. Against Haagensen's advice, Turner decided to take a chance with Revici's treatment, particularly since Haagensen had indicated that there was nothing more that could be done for her.

By the time she arrived at the IAB on May 31, 1964 to see Dr. Revici for treatment, her cancer completely filled one of her breasts and partially filled the other. During her therapy with Revici, a biopsy was performed which confirmed the presence of a scirrhous carcinoma—a fast-growing cancer that also happens to be the most common form of breast cancer. Meanwhile, as with other patients, Lyall and Schwartz would repeatedly try to discourage Turner from the program, telling her, "that she was wasting her time," according to Fishbein.

By January of 1965, the month following the end of the study, Turner went to Dr. Haagensen's office for another breast exam. According to a letter she wrote to Revici, after an initial greeting, Haagensen immediately said to her, "I hear you've been flirting with Revici. He's a quack of the worst kind." Undeterred, Mrs. Turner requested that he examine her anyway.

During the exam Haagensen determined that her left breast was now completely clear of any cancer, and the solid tumor which had completely filled her right breast was both softer and smaller.

According to Turner's letter, in spite of his findings with her, Haagensen proceeded to tell her that he'd, "never found a single person who had been helped" by Revici. When Mrs. Turner's husband asked Haagensen to send a report of his exam to Revici, "[He] refused categorically to send you a report or have anything to do with you." At the same time he "agreed readily" to send the same report to her family doctor, according to her letter.

With the determination that her cancer was completely gone from the left breast and had become much smaller and softer in the right breast, Dr. Haagensen decided that her recovery was due to the removal of her ovaries—a result probably unmatched in the medical literature. The fact that there had been no change in Turner's condition in the four months after her surgery, and that the tumors began to regress only after treatment with Revici's medications, apparently left no impression on Haagensen.

Lyall's response contradicted Haagensen's, but was no less baffling. According to Lyall, scirrhous tumors can shrink over time. When they do so, however, the tumor becomes harder—not softer . Also, they never grow so hard that they disappear, as the tumor in Turner's left breast had done. Haagensen and Revici had additionally found during examination of Turner's breasts that the only remaining tumor had indeed become smaller and softer. Turner's family physician, Dr. Henry Green, confirmed the same results, according to her letter.

Further indications of the apparent bias exhibited by CAG members comes from Dr. Fishbein's January 1965 report. For example, he asks if Haagensen's refusal to submit a copy of his findings to Dr. Revici upon the request of the patient wasn't a violation of medical ethics. In the same report Fishbein also noted the effect of Lyall and Schwartz upon Mrs. Turner:

> She is presently under treatment in the CAG study, but has expressed a desire to avoid any contact with Drs. Schwartz and Lyall because their attitude is very distasteful to her.

Considering the rudeness she had tolerated from Haagensen, one can only imagine the character of the behavior of Schwartz and Lyall.

For at least seven months Turner's case had been accepted as part of the CAG study. According to minutes taken at an Executive Committee meeting of the Medical Board of Trafalgar Hospital in January of 1965, Dr. Lyall told the panel that the Turner case was an example of treatment "failure because of the clinical progression of the disease." The untenableness of that position might have had an effect on Lyall's final decision regarding the case, however. In any case, by the appearance of Lyall's October 1965 JAMA article. his stance changed. According to that report breast cancer cases were excluded due to their "unpredictable growth rates."

According to the protocol, the disappearance of the tumor in Turner's left breast and the tumor shrinkage with softening in the right breast should have been counted as treatment successes.

In another case, a lymph cancer patient named Lucy Hunter was accepted into the study with a tumor which resembled a small red skullcap. The tumor had originated in one of her tear ducts and spread to the top of her head. Cancers that spread to different parts of the body are almost guaranteed to result in the death of the patient. But the patient responded very well to Revici's treatment.

A series of color photographs of her head over a 16-month period shows the tumor steadily disappearing. Yet at the end of the 16 months, Dr. Lyall told Fishbein, "This is a normal phenomena with this type of tumor," and that those kinds of lesions "come and go." Lyle excluded the patient's case from the study, sixteen months after he agreed to accept her case.

According to Dr. Seymour Brenner, her type of case is, "Incurable—nothing can be done." Lucy Hunter was alive and well at the end of the study and continued her treatment.

In the published CAG report, Lyall wrote, "Types of cancer which are notorious for unpredictable growth rates, such as [lymph cancer]... and [cancer] of the breast... were also excluded." The statement was at odds both with the original protocol and with the posture of the American Cancer Society, which recommends early diagnosis and early surgery, chemotherapy, and/or radiation, because if a tumor isn't caught and treated early, it will spread. Lyall's assertion presumes that metastatic breast and metastatic lymph cancer will sometimes reverse themselves. According to the study's protocol, the disappearance of the tumor from Hunter's head should have been recorded as a treatment success.

Another patient who showed rapid progress until he was completely healed, was Mr. Harvey O'Leary. He had a tumor in his rectum that was externally visible. The first photo showed a mass that had the shape of a large bulging oval, red in color, that blocked his anal orifice. The second photo showed a tumor that looked much narrower. The third photo showed the external portion of the tumor to be about the size of an almond—about a third of its original size. By the fourth picture, the external portion of the tumor had disappeared. Physical pressure upon the area of concern by several different doctors indicated that the entire tumor was no longer evident to the touch.

O'Leary responded relatively quickly. Within two weeks of treatment a non-CAG physician by the name Dr. Bruno Sbuelz examined O'Leary and wrote, "[S]ubjectively the patient has no more pain… [the] mass is very difficult to palpate [feel] and [the] dimensions are smaller." Five months later Sbuelz relayed a message from Delafield Hospital to Revici that Herter was also unable to find the tumor. During all this time, Lyall was unaware of the patient. Finally, on March 13, 1964, Lyall examined Mr. O'Leary and claimed that he'd found a tumor of two inches in diameter buried deep in the patient's body. By March 31, Dr. Herter wrote in a letter hand-delivered to Revici by a Dr. Iijima that he had also found a tumor, "with great ease today, and it makes me wonder whether my focus was on the right area."

"Dr. Revici asked Dr. Iijima to show him the mass found by Herter [that day]," wrote Fishbein. Iijima was unable to locate any tumor.

Dr. Schwartz was also present at the institute at that time, so Dr. Revici asked him "to draw a picture of his findings." Indicating that he knew Lyall had reported the presence of a tumor, Schwartz also described a tumor and made a drawing of his findings, at Revici's request.

Lyall, Herter and Schwartz each found a mass with each one finding the imagined tumor *in entirely different locations*, and described tumors of different sizes and with different qualitative characteristics. Herter and Schwartz's exams were on the same day as Iijima and Revici's exam, neither of whom were able to locate any of the tumors described by the three CAG doctors.

All of the various findings became moot one month later when Arthur Glick, M.D., a surgical consultant to the Neoplastic Service of Montefiore Hospital was unable to locate any tumors in Mr. O'Leary.

After all the discrepancies, Lyall had two different responses to the recovery of Mr. O'Leary. While with Dr. Fishbein, Lyall concluded in late 1964 that the tumor was gone after all. According to Dr. Fishbein:

> Several months passed and one day Dr. Lyall told me that he could find no tumor, although a sensation of fullness existed. He said perhaps the tumor had all been removed at the time it was biopsied.

That conclusion contradicted the photographic evidence, however, because the biopsy had predated the series of photos taken of Mr. O'Leary's rectum. It also contradicted his own claim of finding a tumor on March 13th.

Yet in his preliminary report, Lyall told the peer reviewers that O'Leary's tumor gradually grew in size during the course of the study, a finding completely at odds with his remarks to Fishbein as well as the photographic evidence and the physical exams of three doctors, not counting his own examination of Mr. O'Leary which he reported to Dr. Fishbein. According to the study's protocol, the disappearance of O'Leary's rectal tumor should have been recorded as a treatment success.

Despite his own admission of tumor disappearance to Dr. Fishbein, in the published CAG report Lyall wrote, "No evidence of tumor regression was observed in *any* of the thirty-three patients studied." (emphasis added)

In case after case, Lyall excluded patients who appeared to respond to Revici's treatment. Cathy Kramer had been opened up by her surgeon, who observed she had inoperable cancer of the pancreas which had infiltrated her abdominal lining. There were extensive pockets of fluid in her abdomen as well. She also suffered from vomiting of blood. In the post-operative report the surgeon noted that Mrs. Kramer's ovaries were normal. No orthodox treatment was available that could help her. Metastatic pancreatic cancer is quite painful and typically kills its victims within six months, so Dr. Revici decided to include Mrs. Kramer in the study.

Under Revici's care she responded well. Within six months her weight and appetite had returned to normal. "She had freedom from pain or other distress," wrote Dr. Fishbein, who examined Mrs. Kramer with Lyall and Schwartz. Mrs. Kramer's son, who accompanied her to the office, told Fishbein he was confused. According to the son, his mother's surgeon had said he should take his mother home and indicated that his mother might live six months with the care of a nurse. "How, he asked, was such an ominous prognosis consistent with her present condition of good health and normal activity?" wrote Fishbein.

Dr. Lyall decided to eliminate her from the study because fellow CAG member and pathologist, Dr. Arthur Purdy Stout, provided Lyall with a diagnosis of ovarian cancer, a type of cancer that had been excluded from the study's protocol from the beginning. When Dr. Revici attempted to procure the pathologist's report, Lyall tried to stonewall him. Revici then enlisted the aid of Dr. Fishbein to get a copy of the report.

When Fishbein asked Lyall for the pathology report, Lyall responded by saying he was a professor at NYU, and Fishbein had better be careful about crossing him. The threat was not unnoticed by the then vulnerable Dr. Fishbein, who was an underemployed physician recovering from a brain tumor at the time. Fishbein persisted, nonetheless, and obtained the report after several attempts.

The pathology report did little to support Lyall's position and looked to Dr. Fishbein like an amateurish diagnosis. In fact, Dr. Stout's pathology report concluded, "I imagine [it's] a metastasis from the ovary since the patient was a woman and fifty-seven-years old."

Fishbein paid a visit to Dr. Stout at Columbia-Presbyterian's surgical pathology department and showed him a copy of the surgeon's report which stated that the patient's ovaries were normal, "Dr. Stout said that, although he had received the slides [from the surgeon], he was not aware of this information."

Once again, Lyall was not moved by the contradictory evidence. He removed the Kramer case from the study. For purposes of discussion, even if the surgeon was wrong in his diagnosis, and the patient actually did have metastatic ovarian cancer, how many such cases was Dr. Lyall aware of whose prognosis had changed so dramatically for the better? In fact, the prognosis for untreated proliferating ovarian cancer is not much better than it is for pancreatic cancer. Based upon the surgeon's report and the patient's dramatic recovery, the Kramer case should have been recorded as a treatment success.

Furthermore, it is not unusual for research articles to mention promising leads for further study. Lyall made no mention of such a promising lead, if in fact he really believed Mrs. Kramer's cancer was of ovarian origin.

Lyall's strict adherence to a policy of eliminating patients who were diagnosed with ovarian cancer did not apply to Reba Lexington, a 24-

year-old woman with an ovarian cancer that had spread. Because Lexington occupied a bed next to a patient who was part of the CAG study, Dr. Revici courteously introduced her to Lyall. Miss Lexington passed away while Revici was on a trip to Europe.

Lyall told Fishbein he had decided to include Lexington in the study although this ovarian cancer patient had not been a CAG patient while she was alive. Although her case was dropped from the final report, it is clear that the reason for dropping her case had nothing to do with her cancer being ovarian, because he had known that fact all along.

One of the ways the patients were monitored was by directly feeling the contours of the tumor by hand, a process known as palpation. A photographic record would be made by drawing a black line with a felt tip marker around the perimeter of the tumor and taking a picture with a handheld ruler in the picture. To avoid the possibility of bias by Dr. Revici, all of the outlines were drawn by Dr. Schwartz who would then sign and date the photo on the back after the picture was developed.

In one case a male patient with a large belly had a tumor which filled his upper abdomen. Prior to the start of treatment the bottom part of the tumor came within one inch of his navel and extended upward beneath the lower border of his rib cage. In less than six weeks, a second photo showed the tumor had receded upward approximately three inches. Twenty-four days later a third picture was taken. The line drawn by Dr. Schwartz was now a full five inches above the man's navel. Lyall reported in his notes that this patient's tumor slowly grew —a direct contradiction of the photographic evidence. Schwartz, by signing the CAG report, despite his repeated attests to tumor shrinkage in this and in other cases, was complicit as well. According to the study's protocol, the dramatic shrinkage of the tumor should have been recorded as a treatment success.

The conclusion of Dr. Lyall was no less contradictory in the case of an extremely sick Frances Jade. Exploratory surgery performed in April of 1963 indicated she had stomach cancer which extended into her pancreas, small intestine, and parts of her colon. Her surgeon, Dr. Elton Cahow, wrote in a post-operative report that surgical removal of the tumor "was impossible here." Cahow made no attempt to take out any of the tumor. Mrs. Jade died after three months of treatment by Revici. An autopsy was performed in which it was determined that—except for her stomach—the tumor had disappeared. The tumor in her stomach had also shrunk.

Even Dr. Lyall noted in his own summary of the case in his preliminary report that the extensive tumor was limited to a "prepyloric carcinoma" (an area of the stomach) at the time of Mrs. Jade's death. No mention of that admittedly significant reduction of Mrs. Jade's tumor was made by Lyall in the JAMA version, however, although measurable tumor shrinkage was the only criterion for determining the success of the treatment. According to the study's protocol, the disappearance of the tumor from Jade's colon, small intestine, and pancreatic area should have been recorded as a treatment success. The shrinkage of the tumor in her stomach should have also been recorded in the same manner.

One of the requirements of the study was that the presence of each patient's cancer was to be confirmed by biopsy. Lyall did not always follow that requirement. In the case of Mr. Eddie Quayle a biopsy proved to be negative, but Lyall included him in the study after he failed to respond to treatment.

Yet a patient who had no biopsy was excluded. Fishbein told the story of Mr. Rick Samson. Samson got well after a surgeon had previously removed part of a large growth in his ascending colon. Fishbein complained to the surgeon that he was under strict instructions from the patient to perform a biopsy with no other surgery. The surgeon told Fishbein, "[W]ith what he had, you don't have to worry about his recovery. He will be obstructed very shortly." Samson responded quite well to Revici's therapy, however, with no return of the growth.

The Quayle and Samson cases demonstrate Lyall's inconsistency. A patient with a negative biopsy who died was included in the study, whereas a patient with no biopsy, but who was clearly suspected of having cancer based on the surgeon's report, and who was well at the end of the study, was not acceptable. Once again, Lyall made no mention of the Samson case as an interesting area for further research.

A particularly interesting case was that of Mr. Benny Winter. Mr. Winter's liver was enlarged due to a malignancy that had spread from his colon. "The CAG decided to measure the size of his liver at weekly intervals to evaluate the effect of treatment," according to the report written by Fishbein. Everyone agreed that the tumor in the liver had indeed shrunk and grown softer over a period of 14-weeks. Dr. Lyall then decided that the tumor shrinkage was due the general worsening condition of the patient.

Mr. Winter's failure to survive provides a good example of the obstacles confronted when caring for patients whose conditions at the start of treatment are so poor. A lay person might easily be misled into thinking that because the patient died, the treatment must be suspect. But in cases of advanced cancer, there are factors beyond the physician's control, regardless of the quality of the treatment used.

Patients like Mr. Winter are susceptible to all kinds of life-threatening problems. They might suddenly develop internal bleeding. A tumor may perforate an artery or an intestinal wall, which can quickly cause internal poisoning from the patient's waste material. Another major problem is that the patient may be unable to absorb nutrients if the patient's digestive system is damaged. As a result of these and other kinds of problems, shrinking a tumor is only part of the challenge a doctor faces with cancer patients. In Mr. Winter's case, his inability to absorb nutrients prevented him from recovering from his illness.

Every physician experienced in the treatment of cancer knows that a tumor lives at the expense of a patient and grows larger over time at the expense of the patient. Typically it is the patient's overall weight and size that diminish, not the tumor. In those rare cases where a thriving tumor shrinks in size, it becomes harder, not softer.

Nothing in the medical literature would support the conclusion that a tumor that shrinks and becomes softer would cause the worsening of a patient's overall condition. Yet that was Dr. Lyall's conclusion. According to the study's protocol, the shrinkage of Winter's liver metastasis should have been recorded as a treatment success.

Fishbein's report provides an additional clue into Lyall's overall attitude towards the Revici method in the case of Conrad Mann. This young man of 25 years was close to death, suffering from acute leukemia. Every sort of treatment had been tried previously but to no avail in Mr. Mann's case. When he first arrived, he was skin and bones, couldn't swallow, weak, and in severe pain. Mr. Mann's recovery was so spectacular that three months later he returned to work. He was later excluded from the study by Lyall, however, because he had received recent treatment prior to entering Trafalgar Hospital.

In Mr. Mann's case Lyall stuck with the protocol and would not include the patient, although that protocol was more honored in the breach with several patients who did not respond as well. Lyall decided that Mann's spectacular recovery was a case of delayed response to his previous treatments, while Revici's treatment had nothing to do with the recovery. Any readers who are physicians need only consider their own experiences with cachexic leukemia patients who are near death to realize that Lyall's interpretation was entirely singular.

Fishbein mentioned to Lyall how gratified people were by Mann's excellent response to treatment. In return, Lyall inquired of Fishbein, "What sort of hormones have you been slipping to him on the Q.T.?"

A paralyzed cancer patient named Mr. Allen Cantor suffered from extreme pain in both legs. His bronchial lung cancer had spread to his spine. He was given "large doses of narcotics at frequent intervals because of the excruciating pain well-known by cancer patients," wrote Fishbein. The pain indicated that the nerves in his legs were still working, at least in regards to feeling sensation. After barely a month of Dr. Revici's treatment, Mr. Cantor was entirely off narcotics. He reported his pain had decreased considerably in both legs, as he simultaneously regained the ability to move his feet.

Dr. Lyall attributed the loss of pain to increased damage caused by the tumor, a conclusion that is difficult to justify considering the increase in Mr. Cantor's motor function.

To get the full picture of Dr. Lyall's inability to see any benefit in Revici's method, it might be helpful to consider Fishbein's constant presence on the scene. Dr. Fishbein must have cut an impressive swath as a young man with a bald head containing multiple, surgically induced dimples. There he was, with a supposedly deadly tumor that typically incapacitates before it kills, volunteering almost daily, making rounds. Certainly it would have been difficult not to be constantly reminded of the possible efficacy of Revici's method, when day after day and month after month this Yale Medical School graduate continued to show himself in the halls of Trafalgar Hospital not as a patient, but as an attending physician.

It is difficult to imagine that a physician would not be intrigued by the sight of an active young doctor recovering, apparently without incident. Surely most physicians would identify with a fellow doctor's dramatic recovery. That was the setting under which Lyall wrote his findings.

A total of eighteen patients showed measurable shrinkage in the size of their tumors during the course of the study, according to the medical evidence. Oftentimes, tumors shrank to a fraction of their original size, or one or more appendages of a tumor shriveled or disappeared. In some cases the tumors vanished altogether. To the average researcher those kinds of results would have sparked some interest.

In all, eight patients were alive and receiving treatment from Revici at the end of the study. Five of those patients disappeared from the CAG report, however. The other three were dismissed by Lyall as treatment failures, "At the close of the study three patients were under the care of Revici, all showing signs of tumor progression." At least five of the eight were doing quite well, and the other three were improving. At least six of the eight patients were in the terminal stage of their illness when they started their treatment with Revici and all were considered to be incurable, yet they appeared to be thriving in response to their treatment.

As a matter of fact, almost all the patients entered into the CAG study were in an advanced stage of illness, and all of them were considered to be incurable.

There is little likelihood that the eight surviving patients were the result of spontaneous remission. The medical literature reports that spontaneous remission occurs approximately once out of every eighty-thousand cases. In a patient population the size of the CAG, the random chance of eight spontaneous remissions produces a number larger than most calculators can hold. If the ten additional cases of measurable improvement are factored into the calculations, any notion that either spontaneous remission or chance occurrence was responsible for the multiple tumor shrinkages becomes impossible to support.

During this same time period Dr. J. Maisin, who was president of the International Union Against Cancer, of which the American Cancer Society is a member, wrote a series of letters to Dr. Revici expressing how pleased he was with Revici's method. Of twelve miserably ill patients he treated, he found that nine of them benefited measurably and sometimes spectacularly. Revici tried to show Dr. Lyall the results of Dr. Maisin's research, but was rebuffed.

In Rome, Professor Bizru gave a lecture before the Congress of Radiology in September of 1965 where he reported the excellent results he had achieved using the Revici method. Once again, Lyall was not interested despite the original intent of the protocol which was to establish the reproducibility of Revici's work. At the very least, Dr. Lyall should have mentioned the other works and their outcomes.

The CAG report itself was unusual by any standard for the Journal of the American Medical Association. In the front of the article in the upper left-hand corner in bold letters was a two word summary: "Negative Results." The title of the report referred to Dr. Revici by name but not by title despite the fact that he was a member in good standing of the AMA.

Similar to the 1949 JAMA article about Revici, the CAG article reminded readers of Revici's Romanian heritage as well as his emigration from France and Mexico before arriving in the United States. The report also informed readers about the amount of money the IAB had expended as the result of "generous support" from individual and organizational donors.

Like the 1949 report that mentioned the fictitious 52 patients, the CAG report also had trouble with its basic numbers. The report refers to a study that contained 33 patients. Thirty-eight patients were actually accepted into the study. Lyall had unilaterally excluded several patients for reasons such as the ones described above.

In the "results" section of the article, the focus is on the number of patients who died, although all of the patients were expected to die due to their wretched physical conditions when they entered the study. It was Lyall who had originally insisted on excluding mortality or life expectancy statistics from the study. It was Lyall who understood the meaninglessness of counting how many died during the study.

The article also misstated the sole criterion for measuring patient response when it said, "Response to therapy was measured in terms of objective tumor regression *or other clinical change.*" No other clinical criteria beyond measurable tumor regression was acceptable, according to the agreed-upon protocol. (emphasis added)

Lyall referred to the subject of tumor regression on three occasions. In the first case he said in reference to patient autopsies: "In no cases did the examiner find gross or microscopic evidence of tumor alteration as the result of therapy." That statement was, of course, false, as is demonstrated in the cases mentioned above. Revici's critique contains additional examples of autopsy reports that also demonstrate the inaccuracy of Lyall's assertion.

In Lyall's second reference to tumor regression, the report states, "At the close of the study, three patients were under the care of Dr. Revici, all showing signs of tumor progression." Dr. Fishbein provides the names of nine patients, including himself, of patients who were alive at the end of the study. Several of those patients, such as Turner, Hunter, and O'Leary were experiencing tumor shrinkage or absence of any tumor at the end of the study, despite Lyall's assertion to the contrary. Furthermore, Dr. Fishbein is alive today, 33 years after the end of the CAG study, which would indicate that his tumor is progressing quite slowly, if Dr. Lyall's conclusions regarding Revici's method were to be believed.

The third CAG reference contained in the JAMA article more or less repeats the first two incorrect assertions, so it is left to the reader without further comment:

> No instance of objective tumor regression was observed in any of the 33 patients studied; [autopsies] in 15 cases likewise failed to demonstrate gross or microscopic evidence of tumor alteration as a consequence of therapy.

Once Revici suspected that Lyall would not play fair with the results, he made sure that he kept photos of tumor shrinkage for himself. The progress of patients was going so well at the time that Revici convinced himself the final report would be positive, despite Lyall's apparent antagonism.

Revici thought the pictures would protect him:

> In view of the incontestable objective results obtained from even the first cases, from the point of view of the regression of the tumors, I did not want to have the CAG discontinued. I was convinced all the time that no matter how biased or anti-scientific the members of the CAG wanted to be, these results demonstrated through pictures and all the other data, could not be denied.

The evidence would have protected him, if the editors of JAMA had taken notice. When Lyall sent out his preliminary report, Revici responded by sending his own report to JAMA.

While easily understandable to those familiar with the CAG study, the preliminary draft that I located was not reader-friendly to someone who was not familiar with the particulars. But Dr. Robert Fishbein showed me a Revici response that included several groups of dramatic photographs. Even for a lay person, it was clear that Lyall's and Revici's versions of the study were decidedly different. Surely, Dr. Revici would have sent an identical copy to JAMA.

A copy of the Journal's blunt response still survives. In it John Talbott, M.D., editor-in-chief of JAMA, tersely informed Dr. Revici it was not his "duty to arbitrate major differences of opinion." He criticized Revici's submission for not satisfying the basic requirements for a suitable manuscript, and returned it "without comment." Although the Fishbein copy of Revici's report was not suitable for publication, it was more than adequate to demonstrate the false character of Lyall's report.

Copies of pathology and autopsy reports, plus the series of photographs of various patients which Revici submitted, made it abundantly clear that positive results had been achieved during the study. It is difficult to conceive that the contradictions between Lyall and Revici's reports would not have raised a red flag among the editors at JAMA.

Because the medical profession places a high level of trust in JAMA, it is critical that it not publish inaccurate or unfair articles. On the off-chance such an article would slip through the cracks, the onus, it would seem, would be on them to go out of their way to correct any errors. Because the influence that JAMA exercises over the practice of medicine in the U.S. and because lives are at stake, it increases their responsibility and duty to be correct and fair.

There are tantalizing clues as to why Dr. Lyall conducted the study in the manner in which he did. Jon Gregg acted as a liaison between Lyall and Revici during the term of the CAG study. In that capacity, Gregg came into frequent contact with Mrs. Pratt. In her testimony before a state administrative court in late 1984, Mrs. Pratt stated:

> [H]e said to my husband and me, 'You know this isn't going to work. In fact I've even been offered $10,000 to see this fail.'...I never did find out who offered it... but I bet he accepted it.

One internal document prepared by Revici indicates that Gregg's participation was troubling:

> "Gregg told me and made it understood to various persons that everything would be otherwise if he would be continued in his $25,000 a year job. Faced with my categorical opposition, Gregg threatened us with reprisals: 'You will see the hospital and the Institute will be closed. You will be obliged to leave the country etc.'

> "...In looking at the 'aim' of the report, I cannot overlook Gregg's affirmation, in front of Mrs. Pratt, myself and others, that a sum of $10,000 was offered [to] him to write something destroying me."

According to the same document, Gregg, who was paid by the IAB during the CAG study, went to work for Lyall after the CAG study was completed. It is also true that Dr. Lyall wrote a special acknowledgment to Gregg in Lyall's preliminary report: "To Jon Gregg, without whose efforts this study would not have been possible, go our special thanks." He is the only person singled out for thanks in Lyall's preliminary report.

Whether the $10,000 and $25,000 bribery and extortion charges are true will probably never be determined. It is also not evident whether Lyall knew of Gregg's alleged money-raising schemes. Besides, in the end, Lyall's motive is not necessarily all that important. The facts and the records speak for themselves: the evidence is overwhelming that Dr. Lyall was incorrect when he wrote in JAMA, "No instance of objective tumor regression was observed in any of the 33 patients studied...."

Why Revici didn't sue JAMA and Dr. Lyall is an unanswered question. Surely, the cost of taking on a powerful organization like the AMA and its Journal would have been akin to climbing Mt. Everest without oxygen, only a great deal more expensive. The IAB's coffers had been depleted by the cost of the CAG study. (Lyall was paid $20,000; Schwartz $15,000.) Meanwhile, the report itself made fund-raising that much more difficult. The AMA, with its superior resources, may well have played a war of attrition against Revici. Furthermore, Revici was in a position of not having expert witnesses willing to back him up. As demonstrated by Dr. Galbraith and others, there was no future in standing behind Revici in a lawsuit.

Had he sued Dr. Lyall personally, he might have fared rather well. Yet, inexplicably, Revici didn't sue.

When asked, the ninety-eight-year-old Revici would only say, "Lies. Lies. I didn't defend. I could have perfectly sued them." When he said it, he pushed out his lower lip. It's a patented mannerism of his that seems to mean, "I had better things to do." Looking back, it is easy to conclude that Revici made a mistake in not pursuing a civil case against Lyall and JAMA. Yet Revici's interests rarely took him beyond his research or his patients.

Despite the harmful effects of the CAG's false report, Revici continued to see his patients, do his research, and answer his phone late into the night. In the process he made more discoveries, resulting in remarkable treatments for drug addiction and AIDS.

Whether Lyall acted the way he did for money or for some other reason is now unimportant. The good news is that the study conclusively proved that Revici's method was extremely beneficial in the treatment of cancer, even in patients whose illnesses were critical. The readership of JAMA, however, was told the opposite. That discrepancy needs to be corrected. That is, the readership of JAMA needs to be told, in no uncertain terms, of the strikingly positive effects that Revici's treatments had on 18 of the 38 patients.

Despite its falsity, the CAG report clung to Revici like nothing did before. It would later be used against him as if it were the authoritative opinion regarding his work—a legal cudgel to beat him down in a court of law.

29

Magic Bullets for Drug Addiction and Alcoholism Get Shot Down

"That's fabulous! Let's get the rights and give it to Brezhnev."

OCCIDENTAL PETROLEUM CHAIRMAN,
ARMAND HAMMER'S REACTION WHILE IN MOSCOW
UPON FIRST HEARING ABOUT A REVICI INVENTION
THAT COULD CURB THE INTOXICATING EFFECTS OF ALCOHOL.

The effects of drug addiction and alcoholism have left an indelible mark on the hearts and minds of countless families here and around the world. Each time a drug addict or alcoholic is saved, a family is saved. Each time one is lost, society loses. Still, it's a difficult problem to remedy, though many have tried and continue to try. As we have seen from Dr. Casriel's testimony, when a person's steroids are screaming for a fix —reason leaves.

The business side of Revici's drug and alcohol medicines started in a typical fashion for products that possess potential marketability. One of the nation's most prominent law firms specializing in patents, Penney

& Edmonds, represented Revici for a number of his medicinal patents, including the drugs he developed for the treatment of drug addiction and alcoholism. Penney & Edmonds' law partner, Clyde Metzger, brought the medications to the attention of Benjamin R. Payn, Ph.D., a successful businessman who was interested in new technologies.

An impressed Payn struck up a business arrangement with Revici and formed a new company called the Bionar Corporation. Revici had modified the original inventions to eliminate the selenium in a move to facilitate FDA approval. The new drugs were called "Bionar" and "Sobrex". After Revici tested the new drugs, Payn proceeded to work on completing an "Investigational New Drug" (IND) filing with the Food and Drug Administration (FDA). An IND is the first step in the FDA regulatory process. After successfully completing the IND requirements, a drug has to pass several other hurdles before it is finally approved for interstate transport.

Despite the lower costs to perform laboratory tests on animals in the early 1970's, Payn's company spent about $300,000 without successfully clearing the first FDA hurdle. "What would cost a million dollars today to conduct a study on one species of animals, back then cost about thirty thousand dollars, [in large part] because the requirements were less," said Payn. In his elegant Park Avenue apartment, Dr. Payn told me, "If we tested it on monkeys, they wanted it done with rats. If we did rats, they wanted dogs. Mice were done also."

The FDA found numerous reasons to withhold the IND. "In one deficiency letter on Sobrex the FDA listed 10 deficiencies, in another letter on Bionar over twenty [deficiencies were listed]," Payn noted in a correspondence with the author.

While the Bionar company struggled with the many FDA requirements, it did have some good fortune at least on one front. Dr. Harry Simon Levi, a personal friend and trusted advisor to Occidental Petroleum chairman Armand Hammer, learned of the drug and alcohol remedies from his friend Payn. According to Payn, Levi also had a "perfect command of the Russian language," so he often accompanied Hammer on his trips to the Soviet Union.

On one occasion Hammer and Levi traveled to Moscow to meet

with General Secretary Leonid Brezhnev. The Russian custom at some of those meetings included a number of toasts with Russian vodka. Hammer excused himself from the practice by telling his hosts that his doctor's orders prevented him from participating. To avoid being rude to the Russian leaders, it fell upon Levi to carry out the toasts. Hammer saw Levi swallow a capsule and asked him what it was for. According to Payn, when Levi told him it was to ward off the effects of the alcohol, Hammer exclaimed, "That's fabulous! Let's get the rights and give it to Brezhnev."

Payn says Levi countered, "That's crazy. If by an extraordinary coincidence Brezhnev had a heart attack, they'd say the American, Armand Hammer, poisoned Secretary Brezhnev."

Hammer agreed with Levi, but added, "I'm still interested from a business standpoint."

Shortly afterwards, Payn received an unbidden call from an executive of one of Occidental's subsidiaries. "I'm calling you on instructions from Dr. Hammer to find out more about Sobrex," the man said. By June of 1975, the Occidental subsidiary, Hooker Chemical, became a partner in the project. Their entry was none too soon, because the costs of meeting FDA demands had extended beyond the Bionar company's reach.

Hooker Chemical's pockets ran much deeper. Yet, three years of effort by the chemical company brought no better results; the necessary IND could not be procured. In August of 1978 Hooker transferred its interest in Bionar and Sobrex to Continental Group, a multi-billion-dollar conglomerate previously known as Continental Can.

Once again, an all-out effort was made to procure the elusive IND. After three-plus years of Continental's involvement and several million dollars, the IND remained just as elusive. Finally, in 1981, the Continental Group became a privately held corporation. As Payn would tell me in a written note, "After realizing many millions, perhaps ten, had gone into the Sobrex/Bionar project without anything plausible to show for it, the new owners simply gave up on it."

Payn, whose doctorate is in political science, told me, "You can't separate the politics from science. Scientific evaluation was not the only problem. From the best I could tell, some of the scientific staff were strong believers in A.A. [Alcoholics Anonymous]. It was anathema to them that a cure could come from a pill. Also, by then methadone had become very entrenched. It was the only accepted medical treatment for heroin addiction."

Payn recalled one meeting with about a dozen people at the FDA headquarters in Rockville, Maryland. During a discussion, one of the FDA representatives became increasingly angry, "If your thing works, what about a guy who takes several of your Sobrex and thinks he can drink unlimited amounts without getting drunk, and then gets into his car and kills somebody!" Payn tried to tell him the drug was designed for alcoholics to eliminate the craving for alcohol—not to increase its consumption. The FDA representative, who by then had become increasingly angry and red-faced, shouted, "What are you telling me— you call it Sobrex!" Payne said he also noticed a reticence by some FDA staff to consider objectively any drug that was associated with Dr. Revici's name.

With that kind of resistance, Payn and his corporate partners were never able to fulfill the first FDA requirement. Payn likes to point out that an additional cause of the resistance to Sobrex and Bionar came about as a result of the FDA reaction to the thalidomide scare of earlier years. In that particular case an FDA scientist resisted a push to approve the widely used European drug that was later found to cause profound birth defects. The FDA would point proudly to the thalidomide example whenever they were challenged for being too cautious in allowing a new drug to go forward. However, the record shows that resurrection of the thalidomide case by FDA decision makers is not applied equally to all the drugs that come before it for approval.

Hardly a month passes when pharmaceutical companies don't complain about the long period of time it takes to bring their drugs to market. The arduous task means getting an IND and then successfully completing a Phase I, a Phase II, a Phase III, a Pivotal Trial, and a Marketing Application. It normally takes ten years to complete all the steps successfully. Many of those drugs are toxic, some of them extremely so. The cancer drug that allegedly injured Issy received an

IND and was approved by the same regulatory agency that had rejected Bionar and Sobrex.

In contrast, Bionar had previously been used at Trafalgar on more than a thousand drug addicts without any side effects. Both Bionar and Sobrex were designed with non-toxic ingredients. Yet, the combined efforts of the Bionar Corporation, Hooker Chemical, and Continental Group over a ten-year period with several animal experiments and several million dollars expended were not enough to satisfy the "thalidomide" concerns of the FDA.

It is perhaps ironic that while the FDA could not be satisfied with the safety of Bionar and Sobrex, the New York Daily News attacked Revici in its headline for literally using "Sesame Oil." They were right. Perse and Bionar contained sesame oil, a product not considered to be especially dangerous. The FDA has a list of products called, "Generally Regarded As Safe" (GRAS). As a food product, sesame oil would belong on that list. Bionar and Sobrex were made from a fraction of the oil known as a "saturated fatty acid," also a product considered to be safe, much like margarine is considered to be safe.

Whatever credibility the FDA gained by waving the thalidomide scare as its reason for rejecting Bionar and Sobrex, was lost on August 29, 1995, when the Wall Street Journal published a news story that thalidomide had just been approved by the FDA to treat a condition caused by AIDS. Although thalidomide won't be used on pregnant women, the fact that it is a known mutagen has not prevented its approval by the FDA, whereas Bionar and Sobrex have never been found to cause mutations or other toxic effects in any study that was ever performed with them.

With the failure of the FDA to approve Bionar and Sobrex, the United States is left with the addictive methadone as the only medical treatment for active heroin addicts. Methadone is ineffective in treating either cocaine addiction or alcoholism. The little relief methadone has provided in the battle against drug addiction can be measured in inches in that some heroin addicts are now methadone addicts instead. Many would-be methadone addicts have since become cocaine addicts as Dr. Casriel predicted would happen in his Congressional testimony in 1971. Meanwhile, the muggings, robberies, thefts, and murders associated with the drug epidemic have continued to rise.

Methadone's flaws are many and have been discussed by others at length. In short, methadone works by overpowering the patient's steroid levels instead of healing them. The patient is left in an extremely imbalanced state as a result of methadone treatment. Methadone is still used today, but not as much as cocaine and heroin, neither of which, as a practical matter, seem to be much encumbered by the FDA's regulatory constraints.

While the FDA might have helped to prevent Revici's medicine from gaining widespread usage through stalling tactics, others plotted a more direct attack designed to forcibly separate Revici from his patients by revoking his medical license. Little did Revici know that the inaccurate articles of previous years would soon become weapons in an effort to close him down. The Bionar experience demonstrates that sometimes even a couple of conglomerates are no match for the FDA. The next round would throw Revici, a lone physician, against the state of New York, the American Cancer Society, and the FDA.

30

A Two-Thousand-Dollar Pen

"...after all is said and done for the 33 patients,
even if it is shown that the Journal articles are false,
so what?... We believe that by [its] publication in the
Journal it is true, the conclusions are true.

JOHN SHEA, PROSECUTING ATTORNEY,
OFFICE OF PROFESSIONAL MEDICAL CONDUCT

The decade of the 1980's has been, next to Revici's escape from Fascism, one of the most turbulent periods of his long life. In 1983, Revici was slapped with three malpractice lawsuits and an attempt by the state of New York to revoke his medical license.

The dramatic events that transpired during these many legal battles could easily fill a book by themselves. While it would be impossible to tell all the stories that occurred during this difficult time and all the outpouring of support that was provided by the many people touched by Revici's contributions, a few highlights are in order.*footnote on next page

Two days before she died, Cecelia Zyjewski lay in a coma. She had

been semi-conscious for approximately two weeks. Her condition did-
n't prevent attorney Harvey Wachsman from getting her approval to
sue the doctor she loved. Shortly thereafter Wachsman filed a malpractice lawsuit against Dr. Revici in Cecelia's Zyjewski's name. By
mid-December Wachsman changed the suit to be the action of
Cecelia's sister. Later still he changed the plaintiff to Cecelia's nephew.
Wachsman [pronounced Waxman] has never satisfactorily answered
how he was able to obtain permission from a comatose woman to represent her in a civil suit.

It is a serious violation of legal ethics, punishable by possible dis-
barment, for an attorney to file a claim for a client without the client's
permission. Upon learning the details of the original filing, Sam Abady
and Rick Jaffe, attorneys for Revici, would file a motion before Federal
District Judge Mary Johnson Lowe, for a ruling on the matter, to
determine if Wachsman had indeed abused a fundamental legal standard. The judge refused to address that question, however, and dismissed the entire motion.†

On the same day that Wachsman claimed to have become Zyjewski's
lawyer, an NBC Today Show camera crew appeared in her hospital
room to videotape the comatose woman. Wachsman, no stranger to
the TV talk show circuit and a client of a public relations firm, denied

---

* Although the focus of this book has been to inform the reader of the life and travails
of Dr. Revici, I would be remiss not to include Elena Avram. Although her official
title is office manager, Avram has actually acted as the unofficial protector of Dr.
Revici. For nearly three decades she has done everything from raising money, to running the pharmacy lab and rushing to Dr. Revici's side with oxygen during one of his
attacks of pneumonia. She also acted as his pillar during his trying court cases.
Without her efforts it is unlikely that Dr. Revici could have carried through as he did.

† In the original filing of the case, Wachsman's firm purchased an index number which
was stamped on the complaint. After Cecelia died Wachsman's firm improperly purchased a second index number which was also stamped on the original complaint and
which had now been amended to a wrongful death suit. Because Abady & Jaffe were
taking issue with Wachsman's alleged actions in the original suit, they referred to the
first index number. (In fact, it would have been improper for them to refer to the second number because that number referred to the alleged wrongful death suit, and not
the suit allegedly filed by Cecelia Zyjewski.) The judge refused to grant Abady &
Jaffe's motion, however, claiming that the first index number was no longer operative.

he had anything to do with the arrival of the Today Show crew, according to Abady.

The Today Show's Connie Chung presented a dramatic two-part series which portrayed Revici to be just shy of a butcher preying on the unsuspecting sick. The average viewer must have wondered how it was possible that Revici could be allowed to practice medicine. The viewers saw a comatose Cecelia and heard of a doctor whose unchecked actions were a threat to society.

Soon thereafter, three Wachsman clients brought their complaints to the attention of New York State's Office of Professional Medical Conduct (OPMC), which had the power to recommend revocation of Revici's medical license. According to Abady, Wachsman would later deny any role in the simultaneous involvement of his clients in the OPMC action.

The three civil suits of Zyjewski's estate, Edith Schneider and Anne Recce demanded a combined total of $40 million in damages against a doctor who charged his patients about fifty dollars per visit at the time. The lawsuits were the first ever filed against Revici for medical malpractice in his 63 years as a practicing physician. The suits quickly put Revici and his patients in a precarious position, as the combined legal proceedings nearly bankrupted him and resulted in the temporary closing of his practice. The basic facts in each of the three cases illustrate the tenuous grounds for both the civil and the administrative proceedings against him.

Anne Recce came to Dr. Revici for cancer of the breast. Like most patients, she would wait in Revici's jammed waiting room for long periods of time before seeing him. Revici made no appointments, but saw people on a first-come, first-served basis, except that extremely sick patients were given first priority. The waiting room was often a lively communal affair where people would talk about the progress they were making.

Recce was no exception. When she first presented herself to Dr. Revici in October of 1980, she had a hard mass in her left breast that was nearly four inches thick and growing rapidly, according to court testimony. She also had a large, swollen gland in her armpit—an ominous sign. Early in her treatment she insisted on showing her black-and-blue, oozing breast to Evelyn Keisch, another of Revici's patients. An oozing tumor is often a sign of dying tissue, which indicates that the patient is in serious trouble. After a period of treatment by Dr. Revici, Recce saw Keisch in the waiting room again, so she showed Keisch her breast again, only this time it appeared to be normal. That kind of turn-around is unheard of in modern medicine, even today.

During that time the tumor softened and became smaller. In May of 1983, however, after two-and-a-half-years of treatment, she experienced some breast pain. A few weeks later she complained of a severe pain in her back. Concerned about a recurrence of her disease, Revici instructed Recce to get an x-ray. The critical concern was to determine if the cancer had spread to her spine. According to Revici's later testimony to the OPMC, he believed that due to her prior positive response to the treatment, she might continue to do well. He testified, "I have cases of paraplegic [patients] that walk [after my treatment]." The next day Recce's husband came to Revici to get a prescription for some Demerol for his wife's pain. Anne Recce never returned to see Revici, but shortly thereafter she and her husband, who was opposed to the Revici treatment, sued.

According to Revici patient and supporter, Professor Harold Ladas, Ann Recce apparently told Keisch she had gone on vacation and had not taken her medicine with her. It was shortly after that time that her back pain first appeared.

Because after 1978, when Trafalgar Hospital closed, Revici had no hospital in which he could monitor and control his patients' compliance with his treatments. Patients need to check the pH of their urine up to four times a day, take their temperature frequently, and call the office whenever there is a change, either in test results or symptoms. It should be obvious that in a large practice not every patient is going to follow instructions, particularly when it involves constant monitoring day after day and week after week.

For over two years Anne Recce made progress under Revici's care. After she apparently lapsed on her medication, she didn't give Revici a chance to rebalance her system.

A second patient, Edith Schneider, had been to four physicians prior to seeing Revici. Each physician recommended she have a mastectomy performed to remove her right breast. In each case, Mrs. Schneider refused. When she went to see Revici, she didn't tell him that the other doctors had already recommended a mastectomy. She tried to convince Dr. Revici that she didn't have cancer based on an old x-ray. He told her that it was no longer valid and suggested a biopsy. She refused to get one.

In his exam Dr. Revici was the first to discover that Schneider had a second mass located in her other breast. Revici advised against a full mastectomy because of the evidence he had seen that major surgery induces a strong catabolic condition that could easily activate other undiscovered tumors. Instead, he recommended that she have a lumpectomy of the larger mass. She rejected this advice as well. Realizing that Mrs. Schneider was not willing to have any breast surgery, Revici began treating her with his medications on an outpatient basis because he had no hospital privileges at the time. Over the ensuing months she would rebuff Dr. Revici's repeated suggestions that she have a lumpectomy performed. Revici would testify before the OPMC, "[S]he was extremely nervous, bothering me, telephones, and I thought, 'Look, get rid of this. Don't have a mastectomy; have a lumpectomy—only the tumor.' "

Despite her nervousness, she appeared to respond quite well to the treatment. In her civil lawsuit against Revici, a letter was presented into evidence written by one of her examining physicians, Dr. John Castronuovo, which said, "The patient called to say… she had gone to see Dr. Emanuel Revici, and he had given her some wonderful medicine… which had shrunk her tumor [to] one-half of its original size."

After a year the mass in her left breast disappeared, and the mass in the other breast had become smaller and softer. But she apparently panicked for reasons unknown and went to Sloan-Kettering where she had her right breast removed.

The mastectomy apparently triggered a reaction, and a metastases showed up in her left breast soon after. She decided to have her left breast removed as well. Shortly thereafter she and her husband sued.

In Schneider's case, she opted for breast surgery after a year of progress with Revici's treatment. It was Revici's treatment that caused the tumor in her left and right breasts to recede.

For the sake of argument, let us assume that Mrs. Schneider followed Revici's program 100% but still didn't recover from her cancer. That wouldn't make her much different than the half-million people with cancer who fail to respond to their treatment. If doctors were sued every time one of their cancer patients did not respond to treatment, every oncologist in the country would be spending half their time in the courtroom and the other half conferring with their attorney.

The fact that Revici was sued by Mrs. Schneider was certainly not grounds for the state of New York to consider pulling his license. The fact is that most physicians get sued by patients at least once in their career, and many of them are sued several times. Physicians who treat cancer are particularly susceptible to being hit with lawsuits. As a practice the state does not subject them to OPMC hearings as was done to Dr. Revici.

The third patient, Cecelia Zyjewski, came to Revici for cancer of the colon. The large mass occupied two-thirds of the circumference of her colon. During his initial examination of the patient, which took an hour, Revici discovered a large mass in the area of her liver which caused him to suspect that her cancer had probably metastasized.

He also noted that the original tumor was dangerously close to her vaginal wall and may have already penetrated it. (Revici would point out in his testimony before the OPMC that many physicians examining rectal tumors in females fail to palpate such tumors vaginally. This failure sometimes results in an incomplete diagnosis by the physician due to their inability to evaluate the tumor from an anterior [frontal] position.)

Cecelia began seeing Revici on March 25, 1981. At first the treatment brought little in the way of tumor shrinkage, although her pain went away rapidly. After a few months she began to respond quite well; the tumor in her colon had become much smaller. By November 10th the tumor in her colon had nearly disappeared.

Along with the tumor shrinkage, the diarrhea she had experienced for several months without relief also cleared up. Within a couple of weeks of its stopping, she experienced constipation. The change was highly significant and indicated a shift in her condition from catabolic to anabolic. By early December, the tumor could not be located by palpation.

On Christmas day she was admitted to a hospital due to a high fever and dizziness. During her stay an ultrasound of her abdomen was performed. The ensuing report noted, "Examination of the abdomen demonstrates the liver to be normal. After a stay of several days, Cecelia Zyjewski checked out of the hospital and resumed her treatment with Revici. The following March, another exam conducted at Astoria General hospital indicated that "the liver was not enlarged" according to Dr. Philip Levitan, a panelist for the OPMC.

Zyjewski lived with her nephew and her sister, who were both opposed to her treatment by Dr. Revici. The nephew's opposition was so great that Cecelia would call on relatives from another state who lived more than an hour away to take her to see Revici rather than have her nephew take her. According to Dr. Revici, the seriously ill Zyjewski complained to him in telephone conversations that her nephew and sister would take away Cecelia's medicine whenever they would get the chance. Her brother told Revici of the same problem. Once again the ability of the patient to comply with Revici's treatment came into play.

After a year of improvement, Zyjewski's condition began to falter. According to hospital records, Zyjewski was comatose for most of the final two weeks of her life. She was given radiation treatment while there. Dr. Dwight McKee would later testify that the actual cause of Zyjewski's death was an infection resulting from a radiation burn on her back.

Throughout her ordeal, Zyjewski was a loyal patient of Dr. Revici. During one hospital stay several months prior to her death, she called Revici because she wanted to continue his treatment. According to court testimony from her brother and his wife, she supported Revici until the end.

The facts of these three cases demonstrate that none of them provided satisfactory grounds for a lawsuit—much less action by the state to pursue revocation of Revici's license. Had these patients experienced only a temporary improvement before relapse with conventional care, the patients, their families, and their doctors would have shrugged it off as unfortunate but typical. Recce, Schneider and Zyjewski had all experienced significant improvements in their conditions while they were actively following Revici's treatment. From the information available, it appears that for two of them, their condition faltered when the treatment was interrupted. For Schneider, her cancer reappeared after a complete mastectomy was performed, and she had stopped seeing Revici for her care. From these circumstances it would seem that all three plaintiffs' cases had serious problems.

But forces larger than the apparent facts went into motion against Revici. First, Wachsman filed multiple civil suits on behalf of Recce, Schneider and Zyjewski against Revici. At about the same time Dr. David Axelrod, New York State's Commissioner of Health, prodded by the exposure on the Today Show, kicked-off the OPMC proceedings against Revici by suspending his license for 60-days—before the first hearing ever took place—claiming that Revici presented an imminent health threat to the people of New York.

That action created a ground swell of support from Revici's patients who began a letter-writing campaign. Many patients, who feared that they might die if they didn't have access to Revici, contacted Governor Cuomo's office about their critical dilemma.

The first hearing was scheduled in a tiny room at a small hotel behind LaGuardia Airport. About 75 of Revici's supporters showed up for the first hearing. They were told by the panel that the hearing was not open to the public. When the feisty and funny Ruth Spector was told that the hearing was closed she answered, "We'll see about that. Follow me." She opened the door and led the crowd into the room. When one of the panel members tried to tell them to leave, Ruth reminded them, that it was a public proceeding, so they were not leaving. The panelist countered that fire regulations prevented the public from attending.

In the crowd was a maintenance man for the hotel whose cousin had been saved by Dr. Revici from incurable cancer. According to Ruth, he told the panel that space was no problem because there was another, larger room in the hotel that was not being used and that they could shift the meeting to it. The panelists realized that they had been trumped and decided to continue the meeting where they were. Subsequent meetings were moved to a larger room at a Sheraton Hotel in Flushing.

One member of the audience was of particular interest to the panel, according to Ruth. The tall, silver-maned mystery man stood erectly in his black garb. Around his neck he wore a large, ornate cross. Ruth noticed that some of the panelists could not take their eyes off the regal stranger. They appeared concerned that he might be someone of influence. At least one of them whispered to another panelist, inquiring who the charismatic figure was. Ruth didn't recognize him either.

The next day she stopped by Revici's office. The mysterious gentleman was there as well. After they began speaking to each other, the man realized that Ruth didn't recognize him and began to laugh. They had crossed paths three years earlier. At the first meeting, the stranger's appearance was quite different. He had arrived barely skin and bones, folded up in a wheelchair. Shortly thereafter, against the advice of Dr. Revici, he returned on a stretcher to Vatican City to attend an important meeting with the Pope and his fellow bishops. He was the Archbishop of Ephesus, Lorenzo Michelle DeValich.

At the second OPMC hearing, a member of the audience stood up and informed the panel members that if they did not lift the suspension and any of Revici's patients died as a result, they would be held personally responsible and be the subjects of a law suit. The chairman immediately called for an executive meeting of the panel. At the end of their private convocation, the chairman announced that the 60-day suspension was lifted.

The 19 OPMC hearings conducted over a 17-month period contained enough irregularities to inspire a Kafka novel. A few examples should provide the reader with a sense of what was really happening under the cover of a legal pretext.

Carol Flynn, a hearing attendee, was an eye-witness to a comment made by one of the OPMC panelists regarding a medical witness who had traveled from Italy to testify on Dr. Revici's behalf. According to her notarized letter to the Board of Regents:

> In the corridor adjoining the hearing room, immediately follow-
> ing Dr. Ferrari's testimony, I was appalled to observe and hear a
> member of the panel, Dr. Levitan, shouting to someone, 'Did you
> hear him... the last witness to testify... Ferrari? That quack!
> ...[H]e never heard of Bonadonna!' ...Dr. Levitan had chosen to
> disregard all of Dr. Ferrari's statement pertinent to the issue—
> namely the success of Dr. Revici's treatment—and had labeled
> him a "quack" on the single point that Dr. Ferrari was unfamiliar
> with the writings of Dr. Bonadonna.

An attorney acting as the legal representative for the secretive American Cancer Society also provided a window into the tenor of the hearings. During the eighth hearing it became obvious to the Revici defense team that the state was referring to papers in a black box. It is a basic tenet of law that the defense have access to any documents which the state relies upon for its case. Contained in the box were papers that the defense had not seen. The documents belonged to the American Cancer Society. Revici's representative at the OPMC hearings, attorney Henry Rothblatt, demanded that his client have access to the papers, since they were being used to support the charges against him.

At the next hearing, an attorney for the ACS refused to turn them over. After the court had issued a subpoena for the box, the attorney refused to comply. He then proceeded to tell the court that because he was familiar with the papers that were in the box, he would stipulate that there was nothing in them that would pertain to the case. Despite the defense's vehement objections to the groundbreaking legal theory that one side to a case could stipulate for both sides as to the facts of a matter, neither the lawyer nor the ACS ever released the papers to the defense.

On at least one occasion the court allowed the state to question Dr. Revici about a patient without due notice to the defense that the particular patient would be a topic for questioning. As it turned out the so-called patient was actually an undercover investigator for the state. Thomas Flavin had represented himself to Dr. Revici as a person who had been diagnosed as having oat cell carcinoma of the kidneys. He carried a hidden audio tape recorder to tape the appointment.

Because Flavin had brought no medical records with him, Revici refused to treat Flavin and told him that he would need to bring his records before they could proceed. According to a transcript of the tape, Flavin repeatedly tried to put words into Revici's mouth in an attempt to make it appear that Revici would promise a cure. Revici never took the bait, however.

Rather than present the exculpatory evidence that was on the tape which would have demonstrated to the court the extent to which Revici avoided any promise of a cure, the state tried a different tactic. The tactic breached a fundamental constitutional protection which assures that the defendant in a trial be allowed to confront his accusers.

During his cross examination of Dr. Revici, John Shea, the attorney for the OPMC, began to ask Revici about his conversation with Flavin. Flavin had never taken the stand, nor had the evidence on the tape ever been presented before the court. Proper legal procedure requires that the defense be given the opportunity to cross-examine a prosecution witness's testimony before the prosecutor can ask the defense witness any questions regarding it. By skipping over that essential step, Shea placed a presumption in the minds of the panel that Revici had done something wrong, although no evidence had been presented in support of the presumption. Shea asked several questions regarding Flavin's visit —which the panel allowed over Rothblatt's strenuous objections— and placed Revici in a cloud of presumed guilt unsubstantiated by any evidence.

Robert S. Young, M.D., J.D., Ph.D., of the Food and Drug Administration was also brought in by the state as part of its case against Revici. Dr. Young testified that none of Revici's drugs had approval from the FDA, and that in 1965 the FDA had terminated 19 out of 20 IND applications Revici had submitted.

Young would also tell the court that FDA requirements regarding the prescribing of drugs to humans applied only to drugs used in interstate commerce. Nonetheless, Shea expanded the charges against Revici two weeks later by charging him with being in violation of the FDA's regulations.

Perhaps the the most candid admission made at the OPMC hearings was uttered by Shea during the 14th hearing. Revici had started to explain to the panel about particular cases contained in the CAG report to demonstrate its erroneous conclusions. Shea jumped in, "We are not here to prove or disprove the CAG group."

Shea's remark caused the administrative officer for the hearing, Gerald Liepschutz, Esq., to ask Shea, "So you are not claiming that the report is accurate?"

Shea's answer was reminiscent of something out of George Orwell's *Animal Farm*:

"It is not even relevant.... Whether or not it is true or not is not relevant for the purpose of notice."

Liepschutz was a bit perplexed by Shea's answer, so he asked, "How could it be notice of something that might not be true?"

Shea stuck with his circular reasoning:

> The notice, as far as the Journal of the American Medical Association, the Clinical Appraisal Group, the American Cancer Society, is that the method does not work. That's their conclusion.... and after all is said and done for the 33 patients, *even if it is shown that the Journal articles are false, so what?... We believe that by [its] publication in the Journal, it is true*, the conclusions are true. (emphasis added)

When Revici continued to provide the panel with examples of how the CAG report was untrue, the Chairman of the panel, William Stewart, M.D., appeared reluctant to have the cases discussed for the record. He repeatedly asked Revici if the cases were part of the written record already submitted, in an attempt to cut off Revici's testimony. Many documents were submitted during the 19 hearings, including Revici's critique of the CAG report. Oftentimes those documents were the basis for oral examination.

Revici's rebuttal to the CAG report was perhaps the most important document of the entire hearing, for it proved the opposite of what was reported in JAMA—it proved that Revici's method was especially effective in the treatment of cancer.

Because of the critical nature of the rebuttal's findings, it was only appropriate for the panel to focus on them during the hearings. Dr. Stewart's repeated attempts to quash any discussion of the particulars before an audience was not surprising, however.

The crux of the case concerned the efficacy of Revici's method. Yet the panel's concern was whether or not Revici had recommended surgery for the three cases before them. The only frames of reference that the panelists had for judging his method was their own training and the CAG report—which left them poorly equipped to evaluate Revici's method.

If they were to accept that the CAG study actually demonstrated the superior efficacy of Revici's method, the panel would have been forced to agree that Revici's procedures in each of the three cases under consideration were examples of the practice of good medicine. Revici's testimony regarding the CAG patients, which was constantly interrupted by Chairman Stewart, seemed to fall on deaf ears, however. The panel asked Revici a variety of questions that were meant to determine whether he followed conventional medical procedures. In some cases it was a bit like asking him why he didn't use a hand crank to start his car. Because the panel also placed little credibility in the testimony of numerous patients and physicians regarding the effectiveness of Revici's method, the outcome of the hearings was foreordained. Everyone understood that Revici's method was fundamentally different from any other doctor in the state. The panelists had difficulty accepting Revici's unique approach and repeatedly quizzed him on why he did not insist on surgery for each of the three patients. The underlying message from the panel was that any method of treatment outside those community standards as practiced by other doctors had to be malpractice.

In order to provide a cover of credibility for the decision of the panel, a medical witness for the state testified that the Journal of the American Medical Association had published a report (the CAG report) that Revici's method was ineffective in the treatment of cancer and that the American Cancer Society supported that opinion. Accordingly, that information should have informed Dr. Revici that his method was worthless and that continuation of his method in the face of those articles constituted malpractice. That testimony provided the panel of four physicians and one lay person with the justification they needed for their decision.

At the end of the 19 hearings the panel ruled against Dr. Revici and recommended revocation of his license to the Board of Regents. But an odd twist of fate granted Revici a reprieve.

Prior to representing Revici, Rothblatt had enjoyed an illustrious career, and had represented high-profile defendants such as one of the Watergate burglars, the Green Berets, etc. Rothblatt became ill during the Revici hearings, however. He was suffering from a skin cancer which had spread to his brain, but he had kept it a secret. Subsequent court papers noted that he was in a "high state of denial" according to his examining physician. The illness affected his work in numerous ways. He lost files, his speech was affected, his office became strewn with papers, a court date was missed, and he sometimes exhibited erratic behavior in the courtroom. By the last hearing, Rothblatt had deteriorated, so Sam Abady of Abady & Jaffe stepped in to help.

A month after the final OPMC hearing, Rothblatt died. Abady was later able to plead successfully that Revici had incompetent representation due to Rothblatt's terminal condition.

The courts granted Revici a partial new trial, which meant he would be able to present more defense witnesses. This was good news because new expert witnesses had become available to testify in Revici's behalf by this time. Abady and Jaffe had begun to represent Revici in the civil suits as well. This young but talented team looked forward to a fascinating and robust continuation.

But the legal fees to fight the three civil suits and the OPMC trial had long ago exceeded Revici's ability to pay. All along, Revici had depended on the generosity of supporters to pay those bills. As the donors became unable to contribute much more, alternatives were considered. A core of Revici donors decided to hire attorney Tony

Denaro to represent Revici at the new OPMC hearings. Denaro had two major qualifications. While working as an investigator for the OPMC many years earlier, he had exposed alleged criminal misdeeds at that office. Thus, it was believed that he would be a fearless advocate for Revici. His fee was also extremely low.

Denaro's supporters thought his familiarity with the OPMC and its method of courtroom procedure would help. Unfortunately, Denaro had some unusual ideas as to how to represent Revici that backfired and would destroy whatever chance Revici might have had to win over the OPMC panel—or to at least win on appeal. Denaro decided that since Revici's unique method was so unfamiliar to any members of a medical panel that could be drawn together, they were fundamentally incompetent to stand in judgment of his method. Rather than attempting to make his point before the court and informing the panel of the reason for his client's absence, Denaro didn't show up for the first scheduled date of the new hearings.

Denaro would later appeal to the Commissioners of Education (they had jurisdiction in the OPMC case) for an entirely new hearing. After Denaro's questionable strategy was carried out, all five Commissioners were left with little choice but to rule that the state was no longer obligated to grant Revici any new hearings. They also ruled that the earlier decision of the OPMC would stand.

The New York Board of Regents had the final decision on whether to carry out the recommendation of the OPMC panel. Once again, Revici's supporters staged a letter-writing campaign. As a result, the Board of Regents decided by a one-vote majority to place the 92-year-old Revici on five years probation with certain stipulations that he would be required to meet. At the end of the five years they would reevaluate their decision.

After the five years transpired, the board permanently revoked the active physician's license.

• • •

Harvey Wachsman presented a formidable legal foe who liked to travel around Manhattan in a Rolls-Royce. On at least one occasion he made it a point to tell an opposing attorney about a pen he had in his hand, "You see this pen? It cost two-thousand dollars." In addition to his law degree, Wachsman also has a medical degree, although he hasn't practiced since he became an attorney. His law firm of Pegalis & Wachsman specializes in medical malpractice lawsuits. Wachsman likes to say his firm is the largest medical malpractice firm in the country. He is certainly one of the better-known attorneys in that specialty, due to his appearance on Maury Povich's syndicated show and other TV talk shows.

A resourceful character, Wachsman did not limit his offensive to the courtroom. He realized that if the state of New York revoked Revici's license, he could use that as evidence in his civil suits against Revici. He seemed to leave no stone unturned in that effort.

On May 31, 1984, Wachsman testified before a Congressional hearing chaired by Rep. Claude Pepper. The hearing was televised in twenty cities including New York, according to Pepper's introductory remarks. In a letter addressed to Rep. Pepper from Professor Harold and Dr. Alice Ladas, who watched the program in their Central Park West apartment, Wachsman "singled out one physician, Dr. Emanuel Revici, and called him a quack."

The Ladas's also noted, "Wachsman and his clients stand to gain if media exposure pressures the Board into a decision to terminate the proceedings before Dr. Revici concludes his defense."

As Wachsman was surely aware, calling a doctor a quack or a charlatan is considered by most legal experts to be by itself *prima facie* evidence of slander. Testimony given before Congress is exempt from the laws of slander, however.

In the Edith Schneider lawsuit two physicians with ties to the American Cancer Society appeared on behalf of Wachman's client. Victor Herbert, M.D., was one of them. By his own admission, Dr. Herbert had been a member of the ACS Committee on Unproven Methods which he said, "is a euphemism for the committee on quackery."

Although witnesses were not supposed to attend court proceedings prior to their testimony, Herbert, who also has a doctorate in law, sat and observed a defense witness's testimony on the day before he testified. Wachman was also apparently aware of Herbert's presence in the courtroom on the preceding day, but did nothing about it. Herbert came to testify as an expert although the defense had received no advance notice of the witness. When Revici's lawyer, Sam Abady, objected to testimony from this witness whom the defense had no chance to interview beforehand, Judge Constance Baker Motley overruled him.

Court proceedings have an innumerable set of rules to which both sides are supposed to abide in order to ensure fairness. It should be obvious that calling the defendant names of an inflammatory or prejudicial nature would serve to prejudice a jury and make it difficult if not impossible to conduct a fair trial. The judge has the responsibility, if name-calling does take place, to censure the offending party and to instruct the jury that they are to disregard the remarks. If the name-calling is particularly egregious or repetitive, it can be the basis for a judge's determination to declare a mistrial. Witnesses who have legal backgrounds should be particularly aware of the rules against name-calling and inflammatory remarks.

After he took the stand, the legally trained Herbert repeatedly called Revici a quack, saying "We recognize him as a quack.... We consider him one of the cruelest killers in the United States." After Abady's objection to the remarks were overruled, the physician/lawyer, repeated his remark, saying, "We identify in our chapter entitled 'The Cruellest Killers' Emanuel Revici as one of the leading killers in the country."

Besides the inflammatory nature of the charge, Herbert's remark was also inaccurate. Herbert was referring to the 1980 edition of a book called *The Health Robbers*, compiled by Stephen Barrett, M.D. The book is a compendium of attacks on chiropractic, acupuncture, vitamin therapy, and about 20 other therapies, and was written by a number of different authors. The foreword to the book was written by the popular advice columnist, Ann Landers.

The one chapter pertaining to alternative cancer therapies is entitled "The Cruellest Killers." Nowhere does the chapter call Dr. Revici "one of the leading killers in the country" or anything akin to that remark. The two paragraphs regarding Revici provides a very brief description of his theory without making any judgments other than to repeat the CAG report's conclusion that his method was "without value." The paragraph does, however, contain the erroneous statement that Revici's Trafalgar Hospital was closed down by a court order.

Although "The Cruelest Killers" chapter from the 1980 edition of the book lists two authors, in fact the bulk of the article was written by two other authors who aren't listed. The same article with minor differences in wording appeared in an earlier edition of a book also called *The Health Robbers*. The original authors of the chapter both held positions with the ACS and one of them, Lois Smith, is listed in the front of the book as a member of the ACS Section on Unproven Methods of Cancer Management. Prior to her ACS role, she worked at Sloan-Kettering. No mention of the original authors was made in the 1980 edition of the book. The two credited authors of the updated article were also employees of the ACS.

Perhaps the most striking aspect of the article is the lack of substantiation for most of its claims. For example, "The Cruellest Killers" article makes the following unsupported statements in rapid succession:

> Promoters of quackery are often closely attuned to the emotions of their customers. They may exude warmth, interest, friendliness, enthusiasm and compassion.... Quacks tend to be isolated from established scientific facilities and associations. They do not report their results in scientific journals.... Cancer quacks rely heavily on stories of people they have supposedly cured.... Charmed by the quack, however, they believe that his treatment is what helped him.... Many books about unproven remedies are cleverly written so that the reader may think he is getting valuable information when he is not.... Entertainers, politicians and other socially prominent persons are often called upon to promote unproven methods.

The book Dr. Herbert relied upon as his authoritative source as a medical and legal professional to make remarks condemning Dr. Revici was not a peer-reviewed source—rather it was a publication from Dr.

Barrett's own advocacy group, known as the "The Lehigh Valley Committee Against Health Fraud." Thus, Herbert's professional opinion that Dr. Revici is a "quack" and "one of the leading killers in the country" was based neither on science nor a scientific journal, but on the misquotation of an inaccurate article of uncertain authorship.

In his testimony at the Schneider trial during direct examination, Herbert said he was a visiting faculty member "at just about every medical school in the United States and Canada, and at many in Europe." As a visiting faculty member at medical schools across the country, Herbert's influence upon the thinking of medical students is higher than most. Herbert's specialty has been making speeches at medical schools promoting the idea that there is little or no connection between diet and cancer, which presently puts him at odds with the most recent findings of the National Cancer Institute.

Wachsman asked Herbert, "Could you tell us whether the American Cancer Society has any statement or relation in any manner to Dr. Revici with respect to [the committee on quackery]?" Herbert's answer sheds light on why other physicians might be afraid to associate with Revici or to refer patients to him:

"Yes. We identified him in writing as a quack twenty years ago. We have been trying to get the state of New York to pull his license... for twenty years."

The highly trained and influential Dr. Herbert speaks as an authority when it comes to the position of the ACS and its position on quackery. If he says the privately run ACS has tried to have the state of New York revoke Dr. Revici's medical license, he speaks as an insider.

Herbert's reference to "We [The American Cancer Society] identified him in writing as a quack twenty years ago" must refer either to the 1961 or the 1971 "Unproven Methods" articles about Revici which were almost identical to each other. The American Cancer Society's attempt through the state to stop Revici from practicing at the same time that they identified Revici's method as "Unproven" indicates that the term "Unproven" may very well mean quackery in the eyes of the ACS. The desire by this private and secretive organization to see that Revici's license be taken from him might also explain the heavy representation by the ACS at Revici's civil and OPMC trials.

The ACS committee member on quackery then told the jury, "He lies when he claims there is any evidence of efficacy, and he lies when he claims he presents improvements."

Dr. Lawrence LeShan mentioned his experience of repeatedly seeing physicians who were unwilling to risk their careers to study Revici's method. Herbert's enthusiasm in attacking Dr. Revici indicates those doctors might not have been imagining their fears.

Another physician with ACS ties testified against Revici. At the time of his testimony, Dr. Robert Taub held one of seventeen professorships sponsored by the ACS. Dr. Taub said he relied on the CAG report as authoritative because it was published in JAMA. Taub concluded that the publication of the CAG report in JAMA should have put Revici on notice that his method was worthless.

Whether Dr. Taub was a member of the quackery committee remains unanswered. The ACS-supported secrecy of that membership makes it possible for its members to bear witness against a physician without their possible ACS affiliation being known to the court. Taub's presence as a plaintiff's witness, when there are hundreds of thousands of physicians to choose from in the U.S., was consistent with Herbert's statement regarding ACS's desires to have Revici's licence revoked.

In the Zyjewski case Dr. Peter Byeff used the same argument that Taub did, claiming that the JAMA article was authoritative, that it should have put Revici on notice about the worthlessness of his method, etc. In light of Revici's disregard of that notice, Byeff informed the jury that he considered Revici's treatment to be a proximate cause of Cecelia Zyjewski's death. For good measure, Dr. Byeff also testified as to the state of her thoughts during a time when he hadn't spoken to her.

It would be easy to see how a jury, with its faith in the reputation of JAMA and the American Cancer Society would have little difficulty in ruling for the plaintiffs in these two cases.

Revici's own testimony in the Zyjewski and Schneider trials made it even easier. As good as he was as a physician is how poor he was as a strategist and as a witness.

Revici tried to use the trials as a forum to teach the audience about his method. Try as they might, neither his own attorneys nor the attorneys for the plaintiffs had much success in getting Revici to respond to the questions asked of him. In fact, his answers sometimes bore no relation to the questions asked. Embedded in his responses were nuggets of highly exculpatory information, but only someone already highly familiar with his work would have been able to recognize them, disguised as they were in the muddle of his testimony.

To make matters worse, perhaps due the stress of testifying, Revici's command of English grammar was quite poor during his testimony. His English was sometimes unrecognizable, much unlike that seen in his written documents of that time. Tape recordings of lectures from around that time also provide evidence that the stress of appearing in court must have hampered his command of the English language. Regardless of the reasons, his performance was not at all helpful to his cause.

He might have succeeded only in convincing the jury either that he had something to hide or that he was incompetent. According to the candid remarks made by the frustrated judge in the Zyjewski case, the jury quickly lost interest in his testimony. Although the critical remarks were made in front of the jury and were potentially prejudicial against Revici, the judge's comments were quite accurate, nonetheless.

Despite the fact that Revici lost both the Schneider and the Zyjewski cases at the trial level, Wachsman's firm did not prevail in a single suit against him. (The third case, filed by Anne Recce and her husband, was unilaterally dropped before it reached the trial stage.) Attorneys Sam Abady and Rick Jaffe convinced the appellate court in each of the two cases that the patients knew that the treatments they were seeking entailed certain risks, and that they were willing to assume those risks. In its rulings the courts pointed out that patients had a right to enter into those sorts of arrangements.

In each case, the appellate court ruled that the lower court judge should have instructed the jury of that right, and in separate rulings, sent the cases back for retrial. In the Schneider case, which had been argued by Sam Abady, the appellate court stated:

> We see no reason why a patient should not be allowed to make an informed decision and go outside currently approved medical methods in search of an unconventional treatment.... An informed decision to avoid surgery and chemotherapy is within a patient's right to determine what to do with his or her own body.

Dr. Frompovich, writing for *The Journal of Orthomolecular Medicine*, said that the federal appellate court decision in the Schneider case, "May be added to the list of historic dates of individual human rights." In his book *The Cancer Industry* Dr. Ralph Moss referred to the same ruling as "a landmark decision." By its rulings the appellate court, in effect, extended to all patients the same rights that patients of mainstream medicine already enjoy.

Wachsman and his clients walked away from a retrial effort in the Schneider case after Herbert "blew-up" during a deposition. (This was the first time any of Revici's attorneys were able to depose Herbert on Revici's behalf. During the first Schneider trial, Herbert had made a surprise appearance.) As in a trial situation, depositions are conducted while the witness is under oath.

The apparent cause of Herbert's outburst concerned questions by Attorney Richard Jaffe regarding an experiment on folic acid deprivation Herbert had allegedly conducted on himself. It is now known that a severe deficiency of folic acid can cause permanent brain damage. If Jaffe could have elicited from Herbert the possibility that he suffered from brain damage due to an ill-advised self experiment, any jury might question Herbert's status as an expert witness. According to Jaffe, when he asked Herbert about the alleged experiment, "He went nuts."

Herbert also refused to answer any more questions. After Herbert's outburst, Judge John Sprizzo ruled that Herbert would be required to finish the deposition in the presence of a federal magistrate. By the time the deposition was scheduled to take place, however, operation Desert Shield (prior to the Gulf War) had begun. Because Herbert was affiliated with a Veterans' Administration hospital, he was unable to appear for the deposition as scheduled. Rather than approach the court for a new deposition date, Wachsman withdrew Herbert as a plaintiff's witness. Two weeks later the Schneider suit was dropped—eight years after it had been instituted. Herbert never did answer the question regarding folic acid deprivation originally posed to him.

Revici prevailed in the retrial of the Zyjewski case as well. With the case retried in February of 1994, the new jury found in favor of Dr. Revici after deliberating a mere two hours.

Although Revici achieved some vindication of a sort in the civil cases and was able to delay, at least, the loss of his license in the OPMC hearings, it would be difficult to call his ordeal a victory for science, for his patients, or for himself. Certainly his integrity and his dignity remained intact because throughout it all his main focus was the care of his patients. Bob Wilden told me that during that time, "When a sea of chaos seemed to be swirling around him, he was an island of calm."

Still, it would be wrong to think that Dr. Revici was done in by various forces. Revici has contributed far too much to mankind to be measured by the deeds of others. In 1936, when Jesse Owens was competing in the broad jump at the Berlin Summer Olympics, the judges ruled that he had overstepped the line on his first two jumps. As the legend is told, before his last jump Jesse drew his own line several inches in front of the official one in order to dramatically show the judges where he would be starting his jump. Despite the self-imposed handicap, his last jump was good enough to win the gold medal. In a similar way, Dr. Revici has had to prove to his judges that his abilities are above and beyond their abilities to stop him. He has soared and come down a champion.

We are the ones who have been defeated. Sure, there is one office, The Revici Life-Science Center in Manhattan, where his method continues. But that was not Revici's vision—to have a single door to knock on for all the people of the world. His foes have cut off our access to a system of medicine that is far superior to what is presently available. We are the ones who have been crushed, not Dr. Revici. Therefore, it is us—and not him—who must do something about it.

Dr. Revici has spent a century to give the people of the world something for the ages, and someday that gift will be received. It is our choice whether or not we will be among the beneficiaries of his effort.

We can be sure that many physicians would welcome the chance to utilize Revici's method. But as you will see in the next chapter, we should not necessarily expect them to lead the way.

31

"You Will Never Set Foot in Sloan-Kettering"

"Don't use my name."

JOSEPH RANSOHOFF, M.D.,
AS QUOTED BY SEYMOUR BRENNER, M.D.

We have already seen the caution that the eminent neurosurgeon, Dr. Joseph Ransohoff, exhibited in attaching his name to Revici even after he had seen three of his incurable patients make astounding recoveries under Revici's care. Although it would be easy as armchair critics to fault him for his caution, we are not the ones whose career would be put at risk. No matter how well known, there is little future for a lone physician who would attempt to take on the $100-billion cancer industry by speaking in behalf of Dr. Revici. The great weight of potential lawsuits, ostracism, and a team of enthusiastic defenders of the American Cancer Society way of life can make the practice of medicine far more confining than most of us might realize.

We have seen Dr. Galbraith's contradictory behavior of using Revici's method for nine years or more, writing President Eisenhower, and having his wife treated by Dr. Revici under an assumed name— only to turn around and allow his name to appear on the CAG report. Dr. Galbraith was no country doctor. He was president of the Nassau County Medical Society. He also served as president of the New York State Medical Society.

Those were not the only physicians who were touched by the effect of the Revici stigma. Raymond K. Brown, M.D., who worked for two years at Sloan-Kettering, saw it first hand. His assignment was to explore new medical treatments that were outside the mainstream of medicine. As part of that inquiry he arranged for two staff physicians from different medical departments at Sloan-Kettering to go with him one Saturday morning to Trafalgar Hospital on their free time to observe Dr. Revici. But both of the young doctors canceled at the last minute. Both of them were told by their respective department heads that if they went to Revici's office, they would not be allowed to practice at Sloan-Kettering ever again.

As Dr. Brown told Rep. Guy Molinari at the hearing in 1988, "They had been told by the heads of their respective departments, 'If you put one foot in that man's office, you will never set foot in Sloan-Kettering.' " Dr. Brown confirmed to me that each of the doctors separately came to him with the same message. It would appear that the message might have originated from higher than the departmental level due to the similarity of the two excuses.

During my visit to his Manhattan apartment, Dr. Brown related another incident that might provide an insight into the influence that the American Cancer Society tries to use, unbeknownst to the public. Brown said he was shown a letter. It came from Arthur Holleb, executive vice-president of the ACS, on ACS letterhead that was addressed to Robert Good, M.D., president of Sloan-Kettering Institute, which was conducting a Laetrile study.

According to Dr. Brown, the letter informed Dr. Good that Sloan-Kettering's decision to study Laetrile was embarrassing. Holleb invited Good's staff to consult with the ACS before further commitments regarding the Laetrile study were made. Part of the letter appears in Ralph Moss's book. Dr. Brown confirmed that it was the same letter which he saw.

One source, who wished to remain unidentified, said he saw Good's written reply to Holleb, which he described as a "masterpiece of diplomacy." Good informed the ACS executive that Sloan-Kettering was devoted to learning the truth whichever way it led. He also told Holleb that if Laetrile were found to be beneficial, both Sloan-Kettering and the American Cancer Society could rejoice in having another weapon against cancer.

Despite Good's statement to Holleb, his public action was more suited to ACS wishes. According to Moss, the following week Good declared that "at this moment there is no evidence that [L]aetrile has any effect on cancer," despite the fact that early evidence in the Sloan-Kettering lab had demonstrated just the opposite. The studies continued. After several tests conducted at Sloan-Kettering showed Laetrile to be beneficial in spontaneous mouse cancers, and one flawed experiment showed it to be ineffective, the Institute announced that Laetrile was not effective.

According to Moss, Dr. Kenamatsu Sugiura, the highly respected scientist who headed the Laetrile study, flatly disagreed with Sloan-Kettering's official statement regarding Laetrile. Ralph Moss reported in his book that he was dismissed from his job on his first day back to work after he publicly aligned himself with a criticism of Sloan-Kettering's official stance regarding Laetrile.

Dr. Brown had a personal family experience with Dr. Revici as well. In 1971 he took his sister to see Revici because she had developed breast cancer. She was slated for surgery and follow-up radiation treatments. The surgery was postponed for six weeks while she followed Revici's treatment which consisted of daily injections of his medicine.

When the surgery was performed, the excised lump was found to contain no cancer, only degenerated tissue. According to Dr. Brown, after the surgery her surgeon came out and told him, "I'm sorry, something is wrong in the Pathology Department; they couldn't read the specimen. So, I just took her lump out. We'll reschedule her for Monday, when the regular pathology reading comes through." Testifying before Molinari, Dr. Brown went on to say, "On Sunday the doctor walked in to my sister's room and said, 'You have no cancer.' "

As Dr. Brown told Congressman Molinari:

> The pathologist I talked to later said he had never seen anything quite like it. The specimen showed obviously cancerous tissue, but it was all degenerated. My sister knows nothing about medicine, but she said, 'You know it's a funny thing, about a half-hour after I get my shot, I feel a drawing in my breast, on the lump, and also, up on my neck I get another feeling the same way. There's a little spot in my right breast that feels exactly the same; in about a half-hour it pulls and draws.'

When I spoke with Dr. Brown nearly twenty-five years after his sister's treatment by Revici, he reported that she continued to be well, with no recurrence of her breast cancer.

The following example might provide the extent to which the leadership of the cancer research committee has closed ranks against Revici. Dr. Brown provided the author with an exchange of letters with Roswell Park Memorial Institute, a cancer hospital rated by U.S. News and World Report to be the tenth-leading cancer treatment center in the nation.

Because he was acutely aware of the negative impact Revici's name had on the interpretation of any research, Dr. Brown sent a letter to the Roswell Park director, Gerald Murphy, M.D., asking Murphy to test two substances (BNP and TT) for him. Brown intentionally told Dr. Murphy that neither the drug 'BNP' nor 'TT' worked on rat tumors although he knew that they actually did. He also didn't mention that the substances being tested were in fact two of Revici's medicines. Dr. Murphy wrote back rather excitedly, "... although I was told TT did not work in the rat, there are some rather impressive results here due to TT on this tumor in this strain of rat."

Soon after, Dr. Brown let it slip that TT was a drug developed by Revici. The study was immediately canceled. Years later, a letter from

Dr. C. William Aungst, then the director of Roswell Park, was placed into evidence at the OPMC hearings against Dr. Revici. In Aungst's letter, he selectively referred to Dr. Brown's letter to Dr. Murphy in which Dr. Brown stated BNP didn't work on rats,* and left out any reference to the TT medicine.

Dr. Aungst also made no reference to the "impressive results" former director Murphy reported on Revici's TT. As Dr. Brown reports in his own book *Cancer, AIDS and the Medical Establishment*, Roswell Park has since refused to acknowledge that any study with TT ever took place.

The story of one highly recognized researcher might encapsulate why no one is willing to risk promoting Dr. Revici's discoveries. In December of 1989, Professor Gerhard Schrauzer's picture appeared on the cover of *Cancer Research: the Official Journal of the American Association for Cancer Research*. He was also the expert the New York Times went to for an authoritative quote regarding Professor Will Taylor's AIDS research.

To appreciate Schrauzer's standing in the scientific community, I asked another eminent scientist about the former University of California at San Diego professor and researcher. Stanford Professor Arthur Furst, was formerly the long-time president of the American College of Toxicology and a member of the editorial board of *Biological Element Trace Research*. (Professor Schrauzer is the founder and editor of that publication.) When interviewed, Professor Furst, who is also a recognized pioneer in cancer research, commented, "When it comes to selenium, I defer to Dr. Schrauzer. He probably knows more about selenium than anyone else in the world."

Considering Schrauzer's place in the U.S. and international scientific community, I was initially stunned by his remarks in a telephone interview, some of which he would share only off the record. Still, on

---

* The study found that BNP accelerated cancer growth in rats and created vacuoles in the cells. Vacuoles appear in catabolic imbalances. BNP is a catabolic medication and contra-indicated for catabolic conditions. Therefore, Dr. Aungst's negative report on BNP was an unwitting vote of support for Revici's concept of dualism in cancer.

the record, he suggested, in his typically rhetorical shorthand, why Revici has met with resistance from many of his contemporaries: "Revici designed his own drugs decades before anyone else thought of them. Anyone who does this is, therefore, unscientific."

As an eminent researcher with 300 peer review articles published, Schrauzer described the compartmental wall of resistance the medical community has regarding Revici's discoveries, "Even though my own research is in cancer, I am not a physician. Therefore, my advocacy is meaningless."

Despite Schrauzer's trepidations about speaking freely on Revici's behalf, the reader will recall that it was Schrauzer who compared Revici to Hippocrates, Galen and Paracelsus. Schrauzer expanded on that comparison by recalling that Paracelsus was forced to flee for his safety more than once because he made his own medicines, "It was the pharmacists who were after him."

One physician who suffered as a result of conducting studies on Revici's method was Leonard B. Goldman, M.D., a busy radiologist. In a letter written to the New York Board of Regents in January of 1986, Dr. Goldman said he became interested in Revici's work in the early 1950's. One of his former patients had responded spectacularly to Revici's method of treatment. Goldman visited a hospital where he saw other Revici cancer patients, "Many of whom seemed better and were off their opiates."

Dr. Goldman received permission from Revici to conduct his own study with Revici's assistance. In the letter, he reported that a patient had a tumor that had put a hole in her skull, "[It] disappeared, and she was able to become active again." Goldman presented his findings with his own patients at an AMA meeting. "The only result was the suspension of my residency program at Queens General Hospital," Goldman informed the Regents in 1986.

We have already seen that Dr. John Heller was afraid of losing his job as the medical director of Sloan-Kettering if he were to suggest using Revici's medicines at that elite cancer center. His concern would indicate that the resistance to Revici's method came from the top of Sloan-Kettering.

The tentacles of intimidation reach into many different areas. At the OPMC hearings, one of the hearing officers was overheard by Ruth Spector to threaten Dwight McKee, M.D., who worked with Dr. Revici at the time. "We know who you are. We'll get you," the panelist was heard to say. Dr. McKee recently verified the incident in a telephone interview and added that the remark, "Had a threatening overtone to it."

Dr. Seymour Brenner was not totally immune either. He informed me during a visit to his home in Florida that when he began to investigate the case histories of some of Revici's patients, calls were made to the hospital where he was affiliated questioning his competence. His comments echoed his 1988 testimony before Rep. Guy Molinari:

> Now I must tell you briefly my name has already surfaced, and one of the hospitals that I've been associated with has already been questioned by the State as to whether I'm a qualified doctor, and how come a doctor like me is on the staff.

Brenner also reported during the Molinari hearing that when he talked to his fellow doctors about his research, they warned him, "Brenner, what are you doing? You're going to get into trouble."

All of the above stories are the result of this amateur investigator's solitary research with limited resources into the Revici story. The possibility exists that these stories are but a small part of a larger story with the same theme. It is not known how many other conversations have taken place that were variations on that theme. We do know that key players are afraid to act in Revici's behalf for non-medical reasons. It is also clear that the political climate of persecution and closed-mindedness within the medical industry is fixed in its determination to prevent you and me from benefiting from Revici's real medicine.

Individual medical practitioners have been unable to overcome the forces that control the fate of Dr. Revici's medicines. Whether it be the state, the ACS, JAMA, the Lehigh Valley Committee Against Health Fraud, or Dr. Victor Herbert, it is evident that the opponents of Dr. Revici are well funded. Confronted by powers much greater than any lone physician is equipped to take on, it is exceedingly difficult for any one of them to march triumphantly for Revici's cause. Yet, they are kept silent at our peril.

Despite these long odds, over the years a few physicians could always be found to stick their necks out. It hasn't been enough to declare victory, but it has been enough to keep the promise alive, or at least to keep it barely breathing. You have already heard about quite a few of them. The next chapter will introduce you to a few more who have popped their heads out of the fox hole.

32

"Wow!"

*"I've seen the case reports;
I agree with what Dr. Brenner says."*

RUDY FALK, M.D., DIRECTOR OF SURGICAL ONCOLOGY,
TORONTO GENERAL HOSPITAL, MARCH 18, 1988

On March 18, 1988, a lone Congressman held a day-long hearing in order to learn more about Dr. Revici's therapies. Thirteen patients and four physicians came forward to tell Representative Guy Molinari about the positive results Dr. Revici had achieved, either for themselves or for their patients. Author and radio commentator Gary Null, two attorneys, and others also came forward to support Dr. Revici. A dozen letters of support were submitted into the record as well. Only Harvey Wachsman dissented. Wachsman's remarks aside, each person's testimony provided dramatic evidence that Dr. Revici was helping people with his medicines.

For example, Dr. Rudy Falk, Director of Surgical Oncology at Toronto General Hospital and a highly regarded cancer specialist, appeared at the hearing. At the time of his testimony, Dr. Falk had already authored 155 articles published in peer-review journals. In his testimony he directly corroborated Dr. Seymour Brenner's findings concerning Revici's patients: "I've seen the case reports. I agree with what Dr. Brenner says."

Brenner told a story about Joseph Ransohoff, M.D. Among his many accomplishments, Dr. Ransohoff was invited by Roy Selby, M.D., to be interviewed on videotape for the purpose of being included in the archives of the American Association of Neurosurgeons. According to Dr. Selby, that type of invitation is reserved for very select company.

As you have discovered in Part III, Dr. Ransohoff had performed surgery on three patients who ended up in Revici's office. When the first patient told Ransohoff she was going to see Revici, he was not pleased. According to Brenner's testimony the patient told him that Ransohoff said, "Oh, if you're going to that quack, I want nothing further to do with you."

But to his credit, Ransohoff changed his mind, at least privately, when presented with more evidence. Brenner sent him a letter inquiring about the three patients. He told Congressman Molinari, "So, what I did was, I was playing it rather cool." Brenner told Molinari that in his letter to Dr. Ransohoff, he wrote, "Three of your patients were here, and I did CAT scans on them. They gave me histories that they had malignant brain tumors. Could you give me the information as to whether they really know what's wrong with them?"

Brenner testified, "He sent me a letter. The opening sentence is 'Wow! This is amazing. Keep in touch with me.' "

A couple of weeks later a physician came to Brenner for a diagnostic work up and eventually found out he had a highly malignant brain tumor. Brenner sent him to Ransohoff. After a couple of weeks, Brenner called Ransohoff, "What do you think about him going to Revici? He said, 'I agree totally. I'll cooperate in any way I can. Don't use my name.' "

Seven years after Brenner's testimony, Ransohoff confirmed Brenner's account, "I probably did write that, if he said I did." He went on to say, "If Dr. Brenner has documented that some of these people that he has shown me the films on that they were malignant tumors, and the patients were doing very well, that's very unusual."

Ransohoff said he would never discourage anyone from going to see Revici:

> I would never say Revici isn't on to something that was part of a whole new area that's much more respected.... I've always told my patients if we've exhausted what we can do with standard techniques, it can't hurt you if you want to see Revici. Go ahead.

Dr. Brenner also presented his proposal for a major study of Revici's method at the Molinari hearing [See Foreword]. He said federal government approval was needed to begin the study, because the five doctors who would be on the panel would participate only under those conditions.

Gary Null testified about his own experience in investigating Revici's work:

> "I tracked down over 200 of Dr. Revici's cases. I studied this man's work for 15 years. I refused to write an article about him for ten years until I had absolute proof from my own investigation that [these] patients had cancer... it was his treatment that put them into remission, and they were alive and well ten years later.
>
> "Those were the standards I chose before I even announced him to my radio audience. So it's not as if [I'm] someone just running around saying, 'Let's get on the bandwagon.' "

Dr. Revici also testified. His testimony came while his license revocation was under consideration by the state of New York. From Revici's testimony we have yet another indication of his relentless pursuit of medical breakthroughs, regardless of his personal circumstances:

> "I found a method to determine the electrical charge of atoms in the molecule, and I found two atoms with the same electrical

charge bound together. I called them twin formations, and published.

"I looked in the entire literature, and found only one word about it: [Nobel laureate Linus] Pauling telling that this is impossible – it would break the molecule.

"...I went to San Francisco and saw Pauling. I showed him hundreds of different twins, and their importance, because in the treatment I now make, not only in cancer but in general, I utilize largely this concept, because these substances, as I showed, have specific energetic activity."

Gary Null was an eyewitness to the meeting between the two scientific titans. According to Null, after a lengthy discussion regarding *twin formations*, Pauling suddenly sat back, adjusted his famous beret and remarked, "You are now out of my league."

Revici also briefly mentioned another particular area of his more recent research. He had started to identify the relationship between specific metals bound to lipids and their associated diseases. He called these discoveries "Profiles". Revici told the large audience that these Profiles,

...determine for each disease which lipidic element is in charge. [W]e are starting to determine for each individual the specific element involved in deficiency or excess, [in order] to treat him accordingly.

That work could be yet another huge advance in the treatment of a variety of diseases. Regardless of the forum, Revici's focus has remained the same. Although the purpose of the hearing was to put on the record a few of Revici's accomplishments, the inveterate researcher couldn't resist the temptation to share his most recent discoveries. For eight decades his efforts have been directed to helping us feel better when we are sick. His efforts have paid off, even if they have remained largely unknown. In the next section you will see how a few of them can be directly applied.

WHERE DO WE GO FROM HERE

33

Taking Advantage of
Dr. Revici's Research

"Dr. Revici's work is an excellent example of advances in medicine that are far beyond the scope of orthodox medicine."

DR. ROBERT ATKINS, MARCH 18, 1988

Most of Dr. Revici's medicines are made from lipids. The source for many of these products are foods. His medicines are often made by isolating either a catabolic or anabolic lipid from a particular substance such as salmon oil or sesame oil in his laboratory. Because his medicines are made from isolated constituents of the original source, they are quite powerful and should only be taken while under the care of a physician who is knowledgeable about their administration.

That does not mean we must be sick with cancer to benefit from some of Revici's discoveries. Whether it is helping people select the right foods or track their own acid/alkaline balance, some of Revici's

313

findings can have practical applications for people interested in monitoring their own health.

According to Revici, most foods are either mildly catabolic or anabolic. Some foods—like cream, chocolate, sugar and coffee—are strongly anabolic. Fried foods including any type of fried eggs, preserved meat and fish, fermented cheeses, and mayonnaise, are strongly catabolic. In the course of his research, Revici has identified the catabolic and anabolic characteristics of about thirty different types of foods. He has also noted the catabolic or anabolic character of certain vitamins, minerals, medications and other substances. That information might be helpful to readers who wish to choose their foods, vitamins and minerals with an awareness of each one's catabolic or anabolic character. This chapter provides you with a list of some of those foods, vitamins and other substances.

Dr. Revici also comprised a list of symptoms that are often caused by either a catabolic or an anabolic imbalance. That information is provided as well. While it should not be used for self diagnosis, it could provide useful feedback. It is possible to have symptoms from both sides of the list. Usually that occurs when an imbalance at one level of biological organization (e.g. cytoplasmic) causes a defense reaction at another level (systemic).

After examining the food lists below, you might find that your regular diet is composed heavily of either anabolic or catabolic foods. As you review the list, remember that quantities count. If you eat foods from both sides of the list but drink lots of coffee, eat lots of sugar-laden foods, and eat ice cream every day, don't mislead yourself into thinking your diet is balanced.

There are several ways to determine if one is either catabolic or anabolic. One way is to experiment by performing the coffee and soft-boiled egg test. Based both on the demonstration in which Dr. Dudley Jackson experienced no reaction to either an alkaline or an acid drink, and Revici's own experience with patients, a healthy person probably would not notice any significant difference after eating a soft-boiled egg and drinking a cup of coffee. But people who are out of balance might feel either better or worse. Remember, feeling noticeably better is as much an indication of an imbalance as feeling worse, according to Revici's theory.

If you really want to spike your coffee with anabolic foods, add lots of sugar and cream—not milk or creamers from a jar—to the coffee. Be sure the egg is soft boiled or poached—not fried, because fried foods are catabolic. It can be useful to keep a journal to note if there are changes in the way you feel, including any aches and pains.

If you experience a significant increase in pain or a general feeling of unwellness, it could be an indication that the reaction is the result of an anabolic condition. If, following the egg and coffee, you notice a decrease in a pain you already had, that means the pain is catabolic in nature, according to Dr. Revici. In either case you might want to observe how other foods affect you to see if their catabolic or their anabolic nature produces similar effects. Continue to keep a diary of the foods you eat and how you feel shortly after eating them.

After a few days, review your journal to see if you can ascertain whether catabolic or anabolic foods cause discomfort. Also, note if certain foods are followed by a reduction in specific pains—or even a feeling of well being.

It is not necessarily recommended that certain foods be eliminated forever, unless you find that a particular food repeatedly produces an increase in pain. Patients under Revici's care for cancer are advised, however, to avoid certain strongly anabolic or catabolic foods depending on the diagnosis.

Another method that is even quicker than the soft-boiled egg test is to breathe into a paper bag for a short period of time, according to Dr. Robert Fishbein. (Warning: Do not use a plastic bag!!) This technique is particularly useful when pain symptoms are easy to identify, whether it be a headache, stomach ache, or even itching. As you breathe out, you will be exhaling carbon dioxide into the bag. Then, each time you inhale, you will be taking in the carbon dioxide. This will result in an acid increase in the blood. As a result of this increased acidity, anabolic (acid) conditions will be temporarily accentuated while catabolic (alkaline) conditions will be temporarily ameliorated.

An alternate way to perform this test is to hyperventilate without the use of a paper bag until the symptoms either worsen or improve. In this case, worsening of the symptoms indicates a possible catabolic (alkaline) condition while an improvement in the way you feel indicates a possible anabolic (acid) condition.

Keep in mind that acid pains are usually worse in the morning and on an empty stomach, and alkaline pains are worse in the evening or after eating. It does not mean that these pains necessarily disappear during the other part of the day; they are just less intense.

The above self-experiments are not meant to substitute for seeing your doctor. *Nor are they tests for cancer.* Rather they can be used as an indicator of either an anabolic or catabolic state. For minor ailments this technique can provide useful feedback. For example, let's say that the symptoms of a particular headache worsen after the paper bag exercise. It could be a cue to eat fewer anabolic foods, especially the ones that are strongly anabolic, and to eat more catabolic foods. Check with your doctor. He might have a specific reason for advising you as he does, especially if you are on medication

Another way to monitor your acid/alkaline shifts is to chart them with the use of pH strips that are available at all pharmacies. Normal urine should be alkaline in the morning with a gradual shift towards acidity in the evening. Dr. Revici's office asks their patients to record their urine pH at 8:00 A.M., 12:00 noon, 5:00 P.M. and 9:00 P.M., but you can get by just using the early and late times.

The pH strips are designed to change color based on the pH reading. Revici uses 6.2 as the average value, which means that the urine is normally slightly acidic. So the key factor in recording the pH is to note whether or not the readings include scores both below 6.2 and above 6.2. In general the morning readings should be above 6.2, while the evening readings should register below 6.2.

The test can be used two ways. First, keep a record for three days to see if your urine pH is stuck on one side of 6.2 or the other. Second, if you become ill, track your urine pH again to see if a pattern develops. It is a relatively simple procedure.

The morning shift occurs at four a.m., so unless you urinate after that time, use the second morning urine to be sure of an accurate reading. The readings will probably vary from day to day depending on your diet for that particular day. The key thing to observe is that there is a general shift in the readings from above 6.2 to below 6.2 as the day progresses. If you find that your urine pH tends to always or almost always be either above or below that figure, see your doctor.

Because I am not a doctor, I can't tell you that constant acid readings or constant alkaline readings are an indication of an underlying illness. It is fair to say that such a condition is not normal. According to Revici's observations, patients who stay stuck in an acid or an alkaline pH urine pattern either are sick or will be soon. Because the pH test is a generalized test, it should not be relied on for diagnosing any particular illness, but rather as an indication of a general imbalance which could be serious, nonetheless.

Let me caution you that none of the home tests are a replacement for medical treatment. On the other hand, it can be useful for your doctor to know this information. If your physician does not find the information to be important, you might seriously consider switching to one who does.

Please note that the urinary pH test provides information at the tissue (extracellular) level. It does not reflect imbalances at the cytoplasmic level. To determine if an imbalance exists at the cytoplasmic level, either a blood potassium test or urinary calcium index needs to be measured. These are tests your doctor can perform.

Revici states that the average value for total blood potassium is 3.8 mEq. A catabolic imbalance would be reflected in scores that were always below that reading. Anabolic scores would always be above 3.8 mEq. Therefore, you would need to have the test performed early in the day and in the later evening. If the readings are both high or both low, then an imbalance is most likely present.

The average score for the calcium index is 2.5. This test would also need to be given in the morning and in the late evening. The scores should fluctuate below and above the average value. If both scores are below 2.5, a catabolic imbalance is highly likely. If both numbers are high, an anabolic imbalance is the probable culprit. If your doctor is open to working with you, he might be willing to go along with either of these serial analyses.

For those of you who have already been diagnosed with cancer, I want to emphasize that the coffee and egg test and the dietary guidelines are not a substitute for medical treatment.

It would also be a huge mistake to think that surgery, standard chemotherapy or radiation therapy, combined with either an anabolic or a catabolic diet, would have any special therapeutic value. Although it won't hurt you to modify your diet accordingly, those medical processes jolt the acid/alkaline balance much more powerfully than foods can correct. If you are concerned about what other people will think if you don't go along with common medical treatment, go right ahead. Based on the poor track record common medicine has with cancer, you won't have to worry about other people's thoughts for very much longer.

Under current laws, if I were to express an opinion that no one should ever consider chemotherapy under any circumstances unless that medicine is lipid-based and administered only with the anabolic/catabolic condition of the patient in mind, some medical board might say I'm practicing medicine without a license. But I can report the results of the lead article published on September 15, 1993 in the Journal of the National Cancer Institute of NIH. In a major study that included almost every type of cancer, the authors found that chemotherapy provided a "durable response" in 3% of all cases. Another 4% of the patients in the study were found to have a "significantly long survival period." That's a lot of vomiting, hair loss and death for very little benefit.

Each person must choose for him- or herself what forms of treatment they will receive. Whatever you decide, perhaps you will find the dietary guidelines useful while you undergo the treatment of your choice.

If you already know that you have cancer, AIDS, arthritis or one of the other conditions mentioned in this book, and you discover that your pH is stuck either in an acid or alkaline mode, it is up to you to decide what steps you want to take—not mine or your doctor's. Remember, it is your life and not your doctor's. If he were trained in Revici's method, he might be able to help you. If he is not trained in

Revici's method, he won't be able to, so there is no point in asking him to do so.

Please keep in mind that Revici's method relies on fractionated lipids that are not water soluble. The demonstration Dr. Revici performed with Dr. Jackson in Mexico was not done with lipids but with an acid solution and an alkaline solution. Those types of products produce a temporary amelioration of pain, but they are not effective in treating cancer. Therefore, don't try to use bicarbonate of soda or some acid solution to try to treat your or anyone else's cancer. It won't work. It might relieve your pain for a brief period of time, but the long term effects from repeated use of these concoctions could be harmful and could act to delay necessary treatment.

If you decide to try the dietary guidelines, check with your doctor about possible drug/food interactions first. Although your doctor or pharmacist should have already told you which foods to avoid, you might ask him or her if there are any forbidden foods due to any medications you are taking.

Should you use the dietary lists below and find that they provide you with temporary relief from pain, so much the better. Let it be a cue to get professional medical attention.

As a footnote, those who are familiar with other anti-cancer dietary regimens, such as the Gerson program and others, will note that some of the foods on Revici's lists are forbidden by the other programs. The reason for this is relatively simple. Most other dietary programs recommended for the prevention and treatment of cancer are based on the premise that an overly acidic diet is a major cause of cancer. In the United States in particular, that approach is often the correct one due to our generally acidic diets. Thus, methods that increase alkaline foods have helped a number of people. However, some of those approaches overlook the potentially dangerous effects of an overly alkaline diet.

Because the processing of foods can often cause a switch in a food's category, this list should only be used for foods in their natural state unless otherwise noted. Food products with more than one ingredient listed on the label, present similar problems in determining their anabolic/catabolic character, which might be another good reason to eat unprocessed foods.

As you examine the list you might notice that some foods considered to be acidic, such as meats and grains, are listed as catabolic while foods considered to be alkaline, such as soy sauce and vegetables, are listed as anabolic. This is because with foods there is not a 100% correlation between catabolism/anabolism and acidity/alkalinity. Therefore, the following lists of catabolic and anabolic substances should not be confused with lists of acid and alkaline substances.

Catabolic Foods	Anabolic Foods
Meats	Dairy
Nuts	Fruits
Bread	Sugar
Grains	Green leafy vegetables
Fried eggs	Poached and boiled eggs
Mayonnaise	Soy sauce
Fermented cheese	Fresh cheese
Any fried food	Chocolate
Cherries	Alcohol
Cranberries	Coffee and Black tea
Pasta	Butter
Sauerkraut	Honey
Sardines	Fresh fish
Tuna fish	Ice cream
Salmon oil	Vegetables
Cod liver oil	Cream
Fish oils	Olive oil
	Safflower oil
	Corn oil

Catabolic Vitamins and Minerals and Elements:
A, D, B_6, B_{12}, Selenium, Magnesium, Calcium, Barium, Strontium, Manganese, Cobalt, Copper, Silver, Silicon, Lead, Sulfur

Anabolic Vitamins and Minerals and Elements:
B_1, B_2, Niacin, Pantothenic acid, Folic acid, E, K, Zinc, Rutin, Sodium, Lithium, Potassium, Chromium, Iron, Nickel, Boron, Bismuth, Fluorine, Chlorine

Catabolic Hormones:
Testosterone, Epinephrine, Progesterone

Anabolic Hormones:
Cortisone, Stilbesterol, Desoxycorticosterone, Insulin

Miscellaneous Catabolic Substances:
Aspirin, Digitalis, Atropine, Quinine, Penicillin, Streptomycin, Aureomycin, Sulfathiozole, Sulfamerazine, Acetophenetidine, Aminopyrine, Antipyrine, Chloroform, Liver extract

Miscellaneous Anabolic Substances:
Codeine, Cocaine, Morphine, Heroin, Phenobarbitol, Pentobarbitol, Caffeine

Surgery—Extremely Catabolic
Radiation—Extremely Catabolic
Chemotherapy—Either extremely anabolic or extremely catabolic, depending on the medication.

The following lists conditions that are sometimes caused by an imbalance of either a catabolic or an anabolic nature, according to Dr. Revici:

Catabolic: Insomnia
Anabolic: Sleepiness, Drowsiness

Catabolic: Diarrhea
Anabolic: Constipation

Catabolic: Fluid retention
Anabolic: Frequent urination

Catabolic: Recessed eyes
Anabolic: Protruding eyes

Catabolic: Slow heart beat, when caused by pathology
Anabolic: Rapid heart beat or change in heart beat (arrhythmia)

Catabolic: Low blood pressure
Anabolic: High blood pressure

Catabolic: Below normal temperature
Anabolic Above normal temperature

Catabolic: Rheumatoid Arthritis
Anabolic: Osteoarthritis

Catabolic: Migraine Headaches
Anabolic: Seizures

Catabolic: Pain worsens after eating and in the late afternoon and
  evening
Anabolic: Pain worsens on an empty stomach and in the morning and
  early afternoon

Miscellaneous Catabolic Conditions: Burns, Cuts and Hair Loss
Miscellaneous Anabolic Conditions: Chronic Viral Disease

Note that morphine, procaine, demerol and codeine are all anabolic substances. Is it any wonder that these pain-killing drugs would have less effect as long-term pain relievers in cancer for anabolic sufferers? Note also that these drugs are typically given after surgery to dull the pain. Surgery is catabolic, so these drugs would provide strong temporary relief in this case.

Revici suggests that patients with anabolic conditions avoid coffee, sugar, cream, soy sauce, chocolate, ice cream, alcohol and table salt including potassium substitutes. Only salts that contain proper amounts of catabolic minerals are acceptable.

Patients with catabolic conditions should avoid preserved meat and fish, fermented cheeses, any type of fried eggs, and mayonnaise for the same reason. A maximum of one alcoholic drink with a meal is allowed for catabolic conditions.

Other suggestions Revici has offered for temporary relief of catabolic pain include a warm bath (it liberates sterols), 40 to 50 drops of soy sauce in water, or lemon juice. Extended hot baths, Jacuzzi treatments, and saunas are not recommended, however.

For temporary relief of anabolic pain, Revici has recommended bicarbonate of soda, two sardines, or mayonnaise. A tuna fish sandwich, mixed with mayonnaise, would provide three catabolic foods together. Adding lettuce would reduce the catabolic characteristic of the sandwich slightly, of course.

Dr. Revici has found the reason large amounts of sodium chloride contribute to high blood pressure: the two chemicals, sodium and chloride, are both anabolic elements that gravitate to the tissue level. High blood pressure is an anabolic condition at the tissue level, according to Revici. Revici notes that potassium chloride is also anabolic and is therefore not a suitable substitute for people with high blood pressure.

Revici conducted a test with rabbits that were prone to develop clogged arteries when fed a high-cholesterol diet. The first group was given a high-cholesterol diet and no salt. Those rabbits developed hardening of the arteries.

The second group was fed a high-cholesterol diet and sodium chloride. These rabbits experienced even more severe hardening of their arteries.

A third group was given the same high-cholesterol diet and a product called Corrected Salt which is made up of sodium chloride salt with a small amount of magnesium and sulfur products (two catabolic tissue level minerals). These rabbits had almost no hardening of their arteries.

The fourth group of rabbits were given regular rabbit food. This group also had normal arteries at the end of the study. Although Corrected Salt was marketed commercially by a small company in Georgia, it is no longer available. But it tells us that we might want to be sure the salt we use has small amounts of the catabolic elements of magnesium and sulfur in it.

Any medical treatment that does not take into account the fundamental significance of anabolic/catabolic imbalances and the body's lipidic defense system for conditions like cancer, can be dangerous. In particular, practitioners of surgery, chemotherapy and radiation treatments do not consider the effects of these modalities on a most basic biological process: dualism. Therefore, patients who rely on those three methods of treatment should realize they do so at their own risk. As for chemotherapy, in fifty years, maybe less, physicians would probably be arrested if they gave their patients the chemotherapy drugs that are now considered standard treatment.

A word of caution: don't be angry if someone you love has cancer, yet he or she won't stop conventional treatments. Each of us learns at our own pace. People have the right to choose whatever medical treatment they want. People smoke, people drink and people do chemotherapy, radiation and surgery. All of us live and die. None of us does either one perfectly. Love them and let them go.

The final chapter will tell you how you can be treated with the method and medicines of Dr. Revici.

34

Real Medicine

"It's not alternative medicine; it's real medicine."

CAROLINA STAMU, M.D.

*"It seemed to me that in cancer there was a similarity
[to the Holocaust], in that so many innocent people
are struck down, and they and their families have to
stand by and impotently watch this terrible thing evolve."*

STEVEN ROSENBERG, CHIEF OF SURGERY
AT THE NATIONAL CANCER INSTITUTE
(INVESTORS BUSINESS DAILY, Nov. 29, 1996)

"A larger measure of public support will be required."

DR. ABRAHAM RAVICH, MAY 9TH, 1955

It might seem rather odd that physicians and patients would need to go into a political arena to talk about medical advances. We are told that the only respectable venue to discuss what works in medicine are the peer-review journals. We are admonished that only physicians are qualified to make medical decisions. Some critics might even say that Congress should first demonstrate that it can make good laws before it gets itself involved in trying to advocate real medicine.

Furthermore, because medical research is a science, it should not bend to the whims of a democratic mob. The strength of science is its objectivity. No tallying of ballots is necessary—the objective results preclude the need for a vote.

But what are we to do when medicine's test tube cracks and bleeds? What protection do we have when the process becomes infected? Do we surrender our rights? Do we roll over and die?

Perhaps there are times when a little Congressional oversight is just what the doctor ordered. For one, it helps to ensure that any dictatorial tendencies might be kept somewhat in check. As the reader has seen, Revici's medicines have not enjoyed the benevolence of medicine's leaders. Under circumstances such as these, it becomes necessary for those outside the medical establishment to become responsible for returning medicine to its true mission, which is to help people get well.

Many thousands of honest and dedicated physicians, scientists, and others have devoted their lives to help make people well. Yet somewhere along the way, due to the imperfections that all humans are sometimes prone to, certain elements of the medical community have temporarily prevented us from having what we all have wanted from the very beginning: real medicine.

Whatever the reasons might have been in the beginning, the bad impressions that the medical profession have developed against Revici's medicines have festered to a point where it is no longer possible for his method to get a fair hearing in the medical arena. As we have seen in Part IV, the culture of resistance and fear is greater than any single medical leader can overcome.

Paradoxically, this author has spoken to several physicians who believe that Revici really has made the discoveries to carry medicine into the twenty-first century. In speaking to these scientists the most compelling aspect that I've noticed about them is their compassion. Of course I don't believe that these few men and women have a monopoly on that virtue. I know of no doctor who enjoys the day when one of his patients dies. Every doctor wants to give his patients the best medicine available.

But it will take more than a lot of doctors nodding their heads in agreement that Dr. Revici probably has some good medicine. Physicians are not free to do what they think is best for their patients. Their hands are tied; their mouths silenced. Well-intentioned laws force doctors to use only the medicines that are approved by the FDA. (I know of at least one doctor who, due to the FDA strictures, won't use Revici's medicines even though he thinks they are superior to what is otherwise available.) State laws also prohibit most physicians from using any techniques or medicines that are outside the prevailing medical standard.

Some of these laws were designed to protect the patient. But now it is clear that these laws have also kept us from getting real medicine. As a result of these many serious shortcomings, some of our leading lawmakers in the U.S. House and Senate have said they want to fine-tune the law. They have said they want to protect the people and allow them access to the medicine they need when they are sick. It is in the best interest of both the doctors and their patients that this fine-tuning take place.

We live in a great age. The disease of cancer has baffled physicians as far back as there are medical records. Yet, for the first time in history, we have real medicine for it. And that is not all. We also have real medicines for viral and bacterial infections, arthritis, schizophrenia and for many other diseases. Like most great things, however, we are going to have to do a little work for it if we are to actually have access to it.

Part of the problem is that the FDA is not set up to search out and identify medicines that can help. Their job is to keep unsafe and ineffective medicines off the market. Unfortunately, their regulations have had the effect of keeping Revici's safe and effective medicines off the market as well.

The first step necessary to receive FDA approval for Revici's medicines is procuring an IND for each compound to be tested. But Revici has patented more than 100 products that he has used to treat patients. A single, successful IND filing for just one of those patents can easily cost several million dollars. Getting final approval from the FDA to launch that drug on the market can easily cost tens of millions of dollars more. (Final approval for some drugs have run as high as $50 to $100 million dollars.)

• • •

On March 1, 1996, the FDA approved the AIDS drug Ritonavir* for use with humans in the record time of 72 days after Abbott Laboratories submitted its application. It can be done. We know it can be done because it was done. However, I am pointing this out not because there is some hope that Revici's medications are about to receive similar treatment. They aren't.

The Ritonavir case demonstrates that pressure can and does change things. AIDS activists are responsible for providing the initial impetus for the FDA's quick action. Yet, for each person in the U.S. who dies of AIDS this year, there are 15 who will die of cancer.

As insurmountable as it may seem, the FDA is not the greatest factor in preventing Revici's medications from becoming the medicine of choice. The real impediment to legalizing Revici's medicines is the incorrect belief that there is no cure for cancer.

Imagine for a moment what it would be like if the facts about Revici's medicines had already sunk into the general public's consciousness. Is it likely that informed members of the public would stand idly by as they watched a family member slowly die in agony? When people find out, do you think for a moment that Revici's medications wouldn't be available from every doctor in the country? There is no group or industry so large that it could stop the stampede that will occur, once enough people know the truth. The great day when the Revici story reaches critical mass is coming. It is up to each of us to determine how long it will take for that day to arrive.

There is a tiny effort afoot to conduct the study that Dr. Brenner proposed [See Foreword]. Dr. A. R. Salman, a former Revici associate who would be the physician who treats the patients if the IND approvals were to come through, has told me that the original intention is to test eight of Revici's drugs.

As of right now, Revici's office has nowhere near the money or manpower needed to jump through the first FDA hoop. Even under a fast

---

* According to the Washington Post, Ritonavir has caused "diarrhea, nausea, vomiting, weakness and tingling as well as disturbances in the body's sense of taste" during trials of the drug.

track FDA program, the IND process is far more onerous than the small office can handle.

Based on past experience, it is not certain that the FDA is going to be all that cooperative. Furthermore, even under a best-case scenario, with complete FDA assistance, there would still be another 100 Revici medications without approval. Without strong evidence to the contrary, the long FDA journey becomes another *de facto* method for keeping Revici's medicines away from the sick people who desperately need them.

Perhaps the FDA process is unnecessary. Although the CAG *report* proved Revici's method to be worthless, the CAG *study* proved that Revici's method was exceptionally effective in the treatment of cancer. Why should it be necessary to conduct yet another study more than three decades after it has already been proven to work?

The FDA approval process is a prime example of our overly narrow criteria for determining what makes a good medicine. If we found a person lying prostrate in the desert, would we wait for an FDA opinion before we gave the person a drink of water? Revici's medicines have grown back bones for the past 50 years. These paralyzed patients have been able to walk again. We needn't be doctors to know that growing back bones is a good thing. Every day there are people lying paralyzed in hospitals whose bones have been eaten away by cancer. Do we need an FDA opinion to tell us it would be a good thing to give them a medicine that could enable them to walk again?

Anyone who would deny the x-ray evidence has no right to call himself a scientist, for a scientist's task is to observe, not to deny. Denial of the obvious is a task reserved for the unreformed cynic. It is rather preposterous to tell the FDA it can't accept the x-ray evidence that goes back to 1948 which clearly shows rehardened spinal bones that had previously been eaten away. It does not take an advanced degree to recognize the new bone growth in those x-rays—any person with eyes can see it. All one needs to do is to read Revici's book. He tells the scientific reader which medicines worked for each level of biological organization. He even points out which products were less effective.

The bottom line is if Dr. Revici has said products x, y and z are effective, and he shows x-rays to support it, can't the FDA give the patient "a drink of water" and issue its approval for the medicines?

As a practical matter, Revici's office has no ability to come up with even the downpayment for the FDA process, much less the total financing of such an undertaking. The cost to garner approval for just a handful of his drugs could easily exceed $500 million.

Instead of $500 million, what is needed is one percent of that, not in dollars, but in people. Five-million people can do more than $500 million dollars. Not convinced? Well, consider this: more than twice that amount was spent on cancer research last year, and the year before, and the year before that. It has not produced a cure or even the scent of one. But five million people spreading the word about Dr. Revici, the doctor who cures cancer, will put his medicines in every corner pharmacy.

How do we get five million people, though? We learned as a nation, a few years back when a forest fire was allowed to burn freely, that a fire doesn't have to start big to become big. A forest fire knows how to grow. No one has to teach it what to do. If we light a few matches (metaphorically speaking), there is a good chance the story will spread like a forest fire.

When Dr. Martin Luther King, Jr. told the world he had a dream, he spoke of much more than race. He spoke of "All God's children." That's us.

Of course, the occasion for Dr. King's speech was to protest the injustice of segregation. At the time, one group of people was making decisions for another. It didn't work then, and it doesn't work now. In fact, Benjamin Rush, M.D., the only physician to sign the Declaration of Independence, warned us over two hundred years ago:

> The Constitution of this republic should make special provisions for medical freedom as well as religious freedom. To restrict the art of healing to one class of man and deny equal privileges to others will constitute the bastille of medical sciences. All such laws are un-American and despotic.

Dr. Rush's prophetic words have come true to our detriment. When Dr. King pushed for integration, he was told by many to wait because it wasn't the right time. Dr. King eloquently answered that plea by pointing out that time was neutral. It could be used to make things better or make things worse.

For the past fifty years or more we have been told to wait, and to wait some more, because new discoveries were around the corner—to wait because advances were being made, and to wait because testing Revici's medicine takes time. We have waited far too long.

We have waited ten years for the FDA to grant a simple IND. We have waited for thirty-five years for the ACS to read Revici's book and to display within the pages of its publications the x-rays of bones growing back. We have waited forty-five years for JAMA to recant its errors and to investigate the potential fraud committed within its pages.

Now they ask us to wait again. If we do, they will surely ask us to wait again and again. We can wait no longer. In 20 seconds another person will be told that he or she has cancer. Why must that person wait? Why must any of us wait?

We must act, if we are to bring the dream to life. Until now, Revici's method has been kept a secret from you. Now that the secret is out, they continue to keep it from you with their laws. But those laws are the kind of laws that Dr. Benjamin Rush warned us against when he said, "All such laws are un-American and despotic."

In 1992, Senator Tom Harkin, a strong proponent for alternative medicine, sponsored a bill that was signed into law to create the Office of Alternative Medicine (OAM) at NIH. Although its intent is good and it provides a platform where alternative modes of treatment can be heard if not listened to, it would be a monumental mistake to believe Revici's method will ever find its way through that office.

The office provides no grant money. Former Congressman Berkeley Bedell is a member of the OAM's advisory council and is also a strong advocate of alternative medicine. Twice he was cured of serious conditions by alternative treatments, one of which is no longer permitted by the FDA. He called the OAM's lack of funding authority to be "a very bad mistake." In one of the OAM advisory council meetings he called the operating procedure of the OAM "a disaster."

Another council member, Frank Wiewel, was so frustrated with the powerlessness of the council, he asked that the committee be dissolved rather than to continue the charade he saw taking place. The same member pointed out that the OAM was approaching its fourth year without appraising a single therapy:

> Now I'm told it will take a long time to put together a review committee, and the review committees are going to have to be with the Institutes [National Institutes of Health] and the Institutes are going to have to do their peer review.... We are going to be sitting around here and we're going to be old and gray and we will be saying, 'Gee, we should be evaluating some therapies some day, you know shouldn't we get around to that?'

One of the former directors of the OAM nullified what little influence the OAM has by unilaterally deciding how its funding would be allocated without first consulting with the advisory committee. The original purpose of the OAM was to support studies in the field where alternative methods already appeared to be getting results. Instead OAM Director Joseph Jacobs redirected all the money it had for that purpose to laboratory studies which might have little or no direct application to alternative medicine.

It is quite natural to assume that the OAM is the answer to making Revici's medicines available. Even Revici's own office believes they now have a path to success if they could just meet OAM, NIH and FDA requirements. This author has had to shake his head in silence when the office manager has had no answer for the question as to how the governmental obstacles will be overcome, other than to shrug her shoulders and say, "We'll see. We'll get an IND." Of course it's not her fault; when I asked her, it was the only path available to them.

Be wary. Those governmental and medical organizations that have stifled Revici's medicines for fifty years are subject to the same pressures that the rest of the medical community is subject to. Although there are a few within the system who are sympathetic, they don't have much clout. One OAM official who asked to be unnamed said he was working under difficult circumstances. With a trillion-dollar industry built on old methods watching over them, is it prudent to believe the FDA, NIH, ACS and others will allow Revici's medicines to walk through the front door? Their acceptance might mean the end to most cancer surgery, most if not all chemotherapy and pain killers, and most radiation therapy.

When medical science can't regrow bones while one doctor can—yet our laws reward the former and punish the latter, it is time to correct the problem. It shouldn't be necessary to go the expensive and time consuming-route to obtain an IND or to please lobbyists at the American Cancer Society, or the editors of JAMA. It is abundantly clear that the medical community is unable to free itself from its self-imposed strictures. Under these circumstances it is necessary for the laws to be changed so that real medicine can be administered without having its practitioners hounded by a despotic medical community.

There is already support from both Democrats and Republicans to act now. Senator Tom Daschle introduced a bill that has support from Bob Dole, Tom Harkin, Orrin Hatch, Charles Grassley, Paul Simon, Claiborne Pell and others. The bill is called the Access to Medical Treatment Act. An identical bill has been championed on the House side by Representative Peter DeFazio of Oregon.

The bill allows licensed practitioners to use whatever treatment they believe will help the patient get well as long as the the patient is notified in writing that the treatment has not been approved by the FDA. It informs the patients that they accept treatment at their own risk. The law also contains several safeguards to protect the public.

First, no advertising claims with respect to efficacy may be made for the treatments. This restriction prevents licensed practitioners from promoting their products or treatments to the public through advertising. The practitioner is allowed to tell his patients what they can expect from the treatment if they decide to undertake it.

Second, the practitioner must not use any treatment that is known to pose unreasonable risks.

Third, the practitioner must notify the Secretary of Health and Human Services of any treatment found to be dangerous.

Fourth, no controlled substances (marijuana, cocaine, heroin, LSD, etc.) may be used.

The bill also allows the shipment of those medicines and devices across state lines as long as they are used strictly "in accordance with this Act if there have been no advertising claims of cure of specific conditions by the manufacturer, distributor or seller."

These restrictions apply only to drugs and devices that have not received FDA approval. Tylenol and Advil would still be featured on TV, and 5-FU and other cancer drugs would still grace the pages of JAMA and the ACS publications, while Revici's medicines would not be advertised at all.

The bill does nothing to usurp the authority of the FDA. Drug companies would continue to demonstrate the safety of their drugs in the same manner as they always have, if they wish to gain FDA approval. At the same time, the proposed bill requires that patients be notified in writing that they bear the risk should they opt for a non-FDA-approved treatment. The law also requires that the patient is made aware in writing that the method of treatment offered is not approved by the FDA, allowing them to make an informed decision as to whether to proceed with the treatment or to choose some other option.

The bill also prevents charlatans and opportunists from trying to make a quick buck through advertising schemes. Without the ability to advertise their medical benefits, both the manufacturer and the practitioner would have little venue for promoting themselves to the oftentimes vulnerable public

The most important feature of the bill is that it prevents the government from having overpowering control over a patient's personal health decisions. In effect, the bill establishes a system of medicine in which doctors and patients can choose whichever path they desire without fear of harassment.

As Sen. Hatch said at a hearing on the bill:

> ...American consumers want the freedom to use products and procedures that improve their health and we cannot always count on the Food and Drug Administration to foster those freedoms.

At the same hearing Sen. Bob Dole, a co-sponsor of the bill, joined Hatch by saying:

While the role of government is to ensure quality, denying access to a treatment that may be the only hope for a patient is not the role of government. ...in a free market system it seems to make sense to make available non-harmful alternative medical treatments to individuals who desire such treatments, without the federal government standing in the way.

Across the aisle, Sen. Daschle added a personal reason as to why he was reintroducing the bill. He told the Senators present that former congressman, Berkeley Bedell, had experienced an "amazing recovery" from a serious condition but that the treatment Bedell used was no longer available due to FDA regulations.

So what can you do specifically to help? There are probably as many different options as there are readers. Let your own imagination and initiative be your guide. Here are a few possibilities to get you started.

In the sixties a group of people road buses into the deep South to help bring an end to some bad laws. They became known as the "Freedom Riders." As a result of their courageous actions, interstate transportation was desegregated. Today we can do something a lot less dangerous. We can become the "Freedom Writers." Let your congressman and senators know how important the Access to Medical Treatment Act legislation is to you. (You might even want to send them a copy of this book.) You can write to them at:

(Insert Congressperson or Senator's name)
U.S. Congress or U.S. Senate
Washington, D.C. 20015

You can call them, too, at (202) 225-3121.

Each of our letters and phone calls can make a difference. Legislators count each telephone call as 75 constituents and each letter, regardless of length, as 230 constituents. This legislation would be a giant step forward in protecting medical consumer rights and would ensure that more physicians would be willing to utilize Revici's method. As the superior results spread, and more patients demand it, more doctors will want to use it. Although it isn't the whole answer, unless this bill is turned into law, we can be sure that Revici's method will eventually wither away and die for a long time to come.

There is another aspect that needs to be addressed. The medical profession has heard only one side of the story for the past fifty years or more. Medical students, physicians and other medical personnel have been bombarded during that time with a constant barrage of misinformation and falsehoods. Medical residency programs typically include weekly free food sessions sponsored by pharmaceutical manufacturers.

Young physicians exposed to the likes of Dr. Victor Herbert might not have the whole story. Most physicians probably need to be retrained. The drug-company-backed JAMA and ACS are unlikely to initiate that task.

We can. Take a few minutes to write a *brief* letter to each of your doctors telling them about this book and suggest they pick up a copy. One or two paragraphs should do the trick. This act is terribly important if we want to see a more rapid shift in physician awareness. We should not blame them for their ignorance. How were they to know that the information printed in JAMA about Revici was false? They had no more way of knowing the truth about Revici than you or I did. It is essential they be given the chance to learn what has been kept from them.

Keep in mind that the reviews physicians might see of this book in medical journals or from so-called health fraud publications may be entirely negative. You can be sure that any mention made by the ACS and JAMA regarding this book will be more of the same stuff they have been saying for the past five decades. Readers will be told that this author is not a scientist, etc., etc., etc.

It is quite likely that, in an effort to deflect the issue from Dr. Revici's patients, either myself or some other side issue will become their central focus. Therefore, it is vital that your doctors hear from you. Many of them will be as dumbfounded as the rest of us when we first learned that there really is a cure for cancer. Some of these doctors want to be free from the strictures they are presently under, but their only source of information is from the medical literature. It is a source they have been trained to trust.

Although not every physician will receive the information from you with open arms—many will. As more of them see the light, it will help to create a climate of change. It will be really important to win them over without blaming them for the present situation. Any resistance they have will come from an accumulation of 50 years of institutionally bred misinformation rather than from nefarious motives.

You can multiply your effectiveness by letting your family and friends in on this wonderful but long-kept secret. They are sure to know someone with cancer, and they can write letters, too. Before we know it, we can be free from the fear of cancer, and physicians will be freer from the the tight hold of an inward-looking medical establishment.

Another important change that is needed is for insurance companies to cover the costs of treatments for people who choose to be treated by the Revici Method. The biggest hurdle is that insurance companies consider Revici's method to be experimental. What they are unaware of is that his method and medicines are superior to and less costly than the treatments the insurance companies are presently paying for.

The average cancer patient incurs anywhere from $50,000 to hundreds of thousands of dollars in medical expenses. Sometimes the expense of treating a cancer patient can shoot up to a million dollars. The average cancer patient also dies, which unfortunately is often the greatest limiting factor upon the expense. In Issy's case the price tag was around $500,000. Joyce Eberhardt's bills approached a million dollars. Revici treated both of them for the price of an appendectomy.

While we cannot expect the average doctor to provide Revici's method for as low a fee as Revici has done in the past, the method and medicines would still be a fraction of the price of complicated surgeries, toxic chemotherapy, and million-dollar radiation equipment.

If doctors using the Revici method charged an average of $500 for an initial interview, $500 per month for telephone counseling, $250 for each of twenty follow-up appointments and $1,000 for medications, in two years the total cost would be $16,100—a mere fraction of the average cost of cancer treatment today. Even with hospital stays added on for serious cases, the costs would still be much less than the majority of cancer cases.

One area the insurance companies should find especially attractive is the avoidance of expensive, risky procedures. These include 24-hour chemotherapy sessions that can damage kidneys and cost $17,500, not including physician fees, and brain surgeries that can paralyze the patient and easily cost $50,000. When the insurance industry realizes that a single, risky and potentially debilitating procedure can cost more than two years of treatment with Revici's method, they should find the Revici Method particularly attractive to their bottom line.

In addition to the high direct costs of surgeries and chemotherapy, those methods carry the baggage of potential harm, as well as the medical malpractice lawsuits that come with it. For example, if Vernon and Judy Morin were to sue Children's Hospital of Philadelphia for the incident where the flushing out of a chemotherapy drug might have been delayed, the price tag for the hospital's insurance company could be quite high. How much the insurer of Dana-Farber Hospital will have to pay for the death of Boston Globe health reporter, Betsy Lehman [see Chapter 27], is a another figure that should make Revici's medicines look quite appealing.

A recent Harvard study indicates that one out of 25 hospital admissions result in a serious accidental injury to the patient. Whether it be the former Playboy centerfold who suffered serious burns on her chest and back when acid was spilled on her while having cosmetic surgery performed around her eyes, or the diabetic in Florida who had the wrong leg amputated, the practice of medicine can be a high-risk endeavor.

Of course medical people are not demons who want to hurt their patients, but it is impossible to place these patients and physicians in close proximity to sharp instruments and caustic chemicals without having accidents. Medical people are subject to the same shortcomings that the rest of us are. It is actually to their credit that more accidents don't happen, considering the deadly substances they work with every day. All that said, an accident ratio of one in 25 has to be unacceptable to the insurance industry. Surely they would be interested in a method that would greatly reduce that risk.

Unpredictable, catastrophic costs are a danger for the insurance industry as are lawsuits for medical malpractice. In fact, the problem has become so critical that insurance companies have pushed for federal legislation to limit the total amount victims are allowed to sue for in medical malpractice cases. Even so, when the number of high risk and complicated medical procedures increases, injuries and malpractice lawsuits will increase in a corresponding manner.

One way to reduce the number of lawsuits is to support Dr. Revici's method because it is inherently less dangerous than many of today's medical practices. If a doctor were to spill a bottle of Revici's medicine on a patient, the cost would not much exceed a dry cleaning bill. For insurance companies, Dr. Revici's method provides a much more predictable approach to risk management, which might be as important as the lower initial cost of the method.

There are small signs that insurance companies are interested in saving money by allowing patients to try alternative methods. Already, Mutual of Omaha sometimes pays for treatment with Dr. Dean Ornish's program for heart disease. The insurance company discovered it was cheaper to send some of their insureds to Dr. Ornish than to pay for heart bypasses, heart transplants, and their accompanying lawsuits. But for the most part, insurance companies just aren't aware of the billions of dollars in savings they can derive from paying for treatment methods like those of Dr. Revici.

It is unlikely that most insurance company executives have even heard of Dr. Revici's method. We can introduce it to them. Call your insurance company and ask them who is in charge of their risk management department and ask for the name of the company's chief executive officer (CEO). Send the CEO a copy of this book with a request that he pass it along to the company's vice-president who is responsible for risk management. If we are to change what gets covered by medical insurance, it will be necessary to get the insurance companies involved. Once insurance companies decide that Revici's method will help their insureds and their profit picture, they might want to become active partners in this effort.

According to Dr. Jurgen Schurholz's July 22, 1994 testimony before a U.S. Senate Committee hearing on the Access to Medical Treatment

Act, 90% of citizens in Germany can receive reimbursement for alternative treatments. At the time of his testimony, Dr. Schurholz had presided for 16 years as one of the committee chairmen for the German Federal Health Agency Commission.

In his testimony Dr. Schurholz stated:

> A survey conducted five years ago reported that 60% of mainstream physicians prescribe medicines we would consider as alternative.... There are no essential prohibitions of any kind to any treatment, and there are no malpractice problems with alternative medicine. Those who have predicted in the 1970's that the public would be harmed, or that they would fail to seek conventional treatments have been proven wrong.

Health care is at the crossroads. On the one hand, there are rumblings that have become louder and louder. Those rumblings tell us that medical care will soon have to be apportioned. In reality it has already started. Under our present system of health care delivery, apportionment cannot be helped because medical costs have become higher than what we as a nation can afford to pay. With a price tag of one trillion dollars annually and climbing, health care expenditures are high enough to lease every adult in the U.S. a Mercedes Benz in perpetuity.

As costs climb beyond our ability to pay, diseases like cancer are increasing *on an age-adjusted basis* every year. That means that the average cancer patient is dying of cancer at a younger age each year. Those two countervailing forces of increased costs and increased sickness do not bode well for the nation.

For those of us who are well today, it should provide a wake up call. During the last century, the medical community has expended trillions of dollars and tried newer and more expensive substances. Yet the path we are on now looks none too promising, either for cancer or for the plagues that might come our way. Ironically, the discoveries made by the minimally-funded Dr. Emanuel Revici are among the most significant in the history of medicine. With them, medical costs would decline while the quality of care would improve.

There is another factor that has nothing to do with money but, rather, with the way we die. We all hope that when we die, it will be an idyllic scene with family gathered around us as we peacefully exhale for the last time. This scene rarely happens anymore. Even patients who die quietly are often so doped up that their death is more like an overdose than a conscious transition from life to after-life. Although the physical processes leading up to dying are not necessarily easy, Revici's patients often die with relatively little, if any, pain. Since each of us will have a dying experience, it would seem that each of us has a good reason to help make sure those medicines are available when we need them.

Revici's gifts are in real danger of being lost, however. Therefore, we must act now. In acting we are faced with a disadvantage and an advantage. The disadvantage is that a force in motion tends to stay in motion. Unless we make a real effort, our despotic state of medicine will continue ever onward. It is a large undertaking to redirect a trillion-dollar industry, and only worth doing because the rewards are even larger.

Our advantage is that applied truth can change even those things that seem to be implacable. When Martin Luther King was a lad, it would have been unthinkable that state-sanctioned segregation would end in a few short years. It would have been even more unthinkable to imagine that the young man's birthday would become a federal holiday. Dr. King realized a simple truth, however — injustice cannot stand. We have a simple truth as well — unnecessary suffering cannot stand. If we apply that truth, the world will gladly follow.

Don't worry about the negative forces that are sure to attack this book. They have been around for a long time, are well funded, and are not going to change their ways all of a sudden. Rather than becoming frustrated by their resistance, let it be a stimulus for further action. They have money—we have something better. It doesn't matter what they say because we know that "bones grow back." The truth crushed down takes root and becomes an oak. Keep watering the roots.

While writing this book several sincere people warned me that my life would be at serious risk for telling the story of Dr. Revici to the public. These people believe that there is too much money involved to let some amateur writer ruin it all. I believe that a healthy nation is worth a lot more than the scraps that can be made off the sick and dying. All of us will be richer by seeing this through. We grew richer when the nation went out of the iron lung business, and we can continue to prosper by curing cancer.

No one is in favor of unnecessary pain and suffering, and we are moved by the sight of seeing another person dramatically recover from a serious illness. By spreading the message of Dr. Revici's work, we are passing along a message that people have longed to hear. It is not a bitter truth but a joyous one—the bones grow back!

Be a Freedom Writer. Do it now. This book has attempted to give the reader a bus ride to a new way of medicine with a fifty-year track record of success. But it is up to you to bring that new day in medicine to light. You can light a fire that will warm the hearts of 265 million people at home and even more abroad. At present, freedom from the pain of cancer by the Revici Method is available in only one place.* It cannot possibly treat all the people who will be diagnosed with cancer, nor should it have to.

To ensure that the method is available to all of us when we need it, action is necessary—not just next week or next year, but now. Call and write your legislators, show this book to your family and your friends, donate a copy to your library, organize, join a cancer action group. Do what you can, and then do some more. Today we have the *most expensive* medicine that money can buy; we just don't have the best medicine. One person's actions can make the difference—yours. Real medicines are here now. It is up to us to make them available everywhere, including from our own family physicians. Let's be a part of history and a part

---

* The Revici Life-Science Center, 200 West 57th Street Manhattan, NY, NY. 10019. Telephone: (212) 246-5122. The office staff is limited. **Please, in the interest of the very sick patients who need to get through, do not call them *unless you wish to make an appointment*. The Center cannot diagnose over the telephone, describe the method, or send materials.** Thank you for honoring these requests.

Continuing the Revici Method is not done without professional risk. Therefore, we must be sure that no entity attempts to interfere with the right of the Revici Center to provide treatment for those who need it. If you hear that it has come under attack once again, please remember that it is also a direct attack on our individual and national health as well. Please respond as you see fit.

of the cure.

At the same time, it is only fitting that Dr. Revici's genius be recognized through some permanent means. That is being done. Because he has carried himself in an honorable manner both in his professional and personal life, it is appropriate to establish an award with a name that would capture those qualities. Therefore, the award will be called "The Revici Honor."*

On September 8th of 1996 at a party which Dr. Revici attended celebrating his 100th birthday, a new scientific prize to be given in his name was first announced to the public.

The purpose of The Revici Honor is to create a mechanism for recognizing and funding meritorious work in the field of medicine, thereby helping to counteract history's tendency to reward the status quo while punishing the truly innovative. Throughout history the norm has been to penalize the true innovators of medicine. This award will help to blunt that pattern by providing the proper recognition to the very ones whose genius has been shunned by the shortsighted majority. At the same time it will help to ensure that Dr. Revici's many discoveries will be remembered and properly utilized.

To help fund this prize, I will be donating 10% of all royalties from the sale of this book for the purpose of establishing this award which will carry with it a cash prize. With this award, we will be able to support and foster important strides in real medicine. You are invited to join me in this wonderful undertaking.

Working together, we can make sure Revici's method and medicines are available to us whenever and wherever they are needed. Just as importantly, by getting involved, you and I can remove the word

---

This book was written independently of Dr. Revici, The Revici Life-Science Center, or any Revici-connected organization. No one connected with the office has reviewed any of the material contained herein. Any errors are entirely the responsibility of the author.

If you wish to get in touch with the author, please write to William Kelley Eidem in care of Sullivan & Foster Publishing at P.O. Box 246; Planetarium Station; New York, NY 10024. Please include a self-addressed, stamped envelope. I look forward to hearing from you. Thank you.

"scare" from the words "cancer" and "AIDS" and so many other life-troubling conditions. With Revici's many discoveries we are already 90% of the way there. It will be up to each of us to take it the rest of the way home.

As we travel that final stretch, it might happen that some highly trained people with respected degrees and titles will ask questions that might have the effect of distracting or misleading the general public. If this happens, there is one simple answer that will help us and them to refocus: "And yet, the bones grow back." When one is looking for hard evidence, there is little that is harder than a bone. It's a joyous bit of evidence, too. You might want to share that thought when you write your congressperson or talk to your doctor, your family and your friends.

The bones grow back.

Appendix A

CHRONOLOGY OF THE LIFE OF EMANUEL REVICI, M.D.

1896   He is born in Bucharest, Romania.

1916–18 Serves in World War I. He is the youngest lieutenant to be in command of a medical brigade. He is awarded a medal for bravery.

1920   Graduates Medical School from the University of Bucharest at the top of his class, summa cum laude.

1921–36 Licensed to practice medicine and surgery in Romania. Maintains a private practice until 1936. Conducts research in major European medical centers including the Pasteur Institute. Makes his first discoveries involving lipids and cancer.

1921–26 Serves on the Faculty of Medicine, University of Bucharest.

1936   Relocates to Paris with his wife and daughter. Continues his clinical research on lipids and pathological conditions.

1937–38 When getting even one paper publshed was a great honor, the Pasteur Institute deposits all 5 papers submitted by Revici on lipids in pathological pain and cancer in the National Academy of Science (France).

1938–39 As his reputation soars, Revici reverses the cancer of the wife of an advisor to the president of France. He is awarded the French Legion of Honor which he declines in order to keep his medical practice free from political influence. Later, after turning over patents and inventions to the French government to aid its fight against the invading Nazis, he is again offered the French Legion of Honor award and again he declines to accept.

1941–46 He is forced to flee to Mexico because of his medical aid to the French Resistance. In Mexico City he founds the first Institute of Applied Biology (IAB). As in Paris, his reputation grows and many physicians from the United States travel to the IAB to observe his work firsthand. He successfully treats the cancer condition of the wife of the ambassador to Mexico from the USSR, then an ally. As a result he is offered the Stalin Decoration by Molotov, along with the sum of $50,000 and the chance to have his own institute in the Crimea. Revici declines the offer.

1946 He is invited by the chairman of the Medical Department, University of Chicago, to forward his research. His entry into the U.S. was facilitated by Sumner Welles, an aid to President Roosevelt, in recognition for his work with the French Resistance and the beneficial potential of his therapeutic methods.

1947 Permanently settles to New York City. Passes the examination for his New York State medical license on the first attempt. Co-founds the second Institute of Applied Biology in Brooklyn, New York.

1948 Invited twice by the U.S. Navy to conduct research on radiation from A-Bomb-test fallout at Bikini Atoll. Receives the highest security clearance. He declines the invitation so he can devote himself to the study of lipids in chronic diseases, especially cancer.

1949 An unexpected setback to Revici's career occurs when the highly influential Journal of the American Medical Association (JAMA) publishes what is later proven to be a fictitious report about Revici.'s methods. Among other things, the report discusses the ineffectiveness of Revici's method while treating 52 "phantom" patients at the University of Chicago. A written FBI report confirmed that Revici never treated *any* patients at the University of Chicago.

1949   Revici meets with Albert Einstein to help formulate a mathematical definition of lipids.

1949   Sues Brooklyn Cancer Society for circulating material defaming him and his associates at the IAB. The suit is arbitrated in favor of Revici. Arbitrator, John Masterson, M.D., president of the Medical Society of the State of New York, becomes a member of the IAB's board of directors.

1950   Reads his paper on abnormal fatty acids (leukotrienes) produced by radiation at the Sixth International Congress of Radiology in London. Revici's paper predates the "rediscovery" of leukotrienes by Bengt Samuelsson who was awarded the Nobel Prize in 1982. Biochemist Barry Sears, Ph.D. bases much of his groundbreaking book, *The Zone*, on the work of Samuelsson. (Revici further discusses these "abnormal trienically-conjugated fatty acids" in his textbook published in 1961, and reprinted in 1997).

1955   Purchases Trafalgar Hospital in Manhattan. Revici becomes medical director and chief of oncology. Relocates the IAB to a site across the street.

1957   Revici wins a libel suit against Kemsley Newspapers, Ltd. (UK). Sir Hartley Shawcross (later Lord Shawcross), attorney for Revici, served as attorney for Sir Winston Churchill and his family (and had been chief British prosecutor at the Nuremberg Trials of Nazi war leaders).

1961   **(March)** American Cancer Society places Revici on its "unproven methods" list.

(July) Revici publishes his major textbook, *Research in Physiopathology As [A] Basis For Guided Chemotherapy.* (D. Van Nostrand). Besides being a lifesaving textbook on cancer treatment, the work details Revici's research-based paradigm shifts, including the theory of biological dualism, the theory of hierarchic organization, and Revici's theory of evolution.

(November) After reviewing his book in depth, The Society for Promoting International Scientific Relations, whose board includes 14 Nobel Prize winners, awards Revici its annual medal.

1965   The CAG report appears in JAMA claiming Revici's method has no effect. One co-signing physician calls the report "a disgrace". Another co-signing physician was secretly so impressed with Revici's work, that he writes to the President of the United States in favor of Revici's method, and has his wife's cancer treated by Revici personally. The report is contradicted by staggering amounts of documented evidence and the written eyewitness account of Robert Fishbein, M.D.

1965   In Rome Professor Bizru gives a lecture before the Congress of Radiology where he reports the excellent results he has achieved using the Revici method.

1965–70 Revici corresponds with Professor Joseph Maisin of Belgium, formerly president and editor of the International Union Against Cancer and world-reknowned as an authority in cancer. Working with terminally-ill patients, Maisin utilizes many of Revici's methods with startling results. The correspondence ends when Maisin dies from a car accident in 1971.

1970   The president of the Medical Society of the State of New York sends Revici an official letter commending him for 50 years of devoted, distinguished patient care.

1970–72 Revici treats 3,000 heroin addicts with two lipidic substances, physically detoxifying the great majority in 3 to 7 days with no withdrawal symptoms.

1971   House Select Committee on Crime holds a hearing on narcotic addiction. Daniel Casriel, M.D. gives testimony on the superior results achieved in the treatment of narcotic addiction with Dr. Revici's compounds.

1972   A feature article in *Barrons* (9/11/72), reports on Revici's amazing addiction treatments.

1977   Revici closes Trafalgar Hospital because of financial difficulty (the hospital had been chartered as a non-profit health facility).

1983-87 After 63 years of devoted patient care, an attorney, representing three patients, files the first negligence suit against Revici. Revici prevails in all three cases. One case, *Schneider vs Revici*, establishes a precedent-setting decision. The U.S. Court of Appeals sees "no reason why a patient should not be allowed to make an informed decision to go outside currently approved medical methods in search of an unconventional treatment".

1984   Edoardo Pacelli, M.D. in Naples, Italy, reports his results with 372 terminal patients using the Revici Method. compared to the results reported with the standard chemotherapy, the results are nothing short of phenomenal.

1988   **(March)** Congressman Guy Molinari (NY) conducts a fact-finding hearing on Revici in New York. Many people testify on Revici's behalf including three mainstream physicians.

(July) The Board of Regents, NY, commutes an OPMC decision, and places Revici on five years probation. The OPMC panel's decision was fueled by the 1965 CAG report appearing in JAMA.

1989   Revici pays a house call to a patient who is too sick to see him, walking up five flights of stairs. He is ninety-three.

1990   The Office of Technology Assessment, an investigative arm of Congress, issues a report on unconventional cancer treatments, including the Revici Method. Seymour Brenner, M.D., board-certified radiation oncologist, testifies to the successful results he has seen Revici achieve with cancer patients.

1990   The IAB ceases to exists and Revici moves his offices to mid-town Manhattan.

1992   Congress creates the Office of Alternative Medicine in the National Institutes of Health (NIH). The OAM and the FDA begin a joint effort to devise a protocol for evaluating Revici's therapy.

1993   Revici's medical license is revoked due to inadequate record keeping.

1996   Revici celebrates his 100th birthday. Accolades come from doctors, researchers, friends, former patients, reporters, and government leaders including Governor Pataki (NY) and President Clinton.

1997   In Zimbabwe the James Mobb clinic reports that protocols developed by Revici are superior to treatments using protease inhibitors, getting wheelcharied AIDS patients back to work in weeks.

1997   At the F.A.I.M. (Foundation for the Advancement of Innovative Medicine) conference in New York, Revici receives an extended standing ovation for his lifetime of extraordinary achievement.

Appendix B

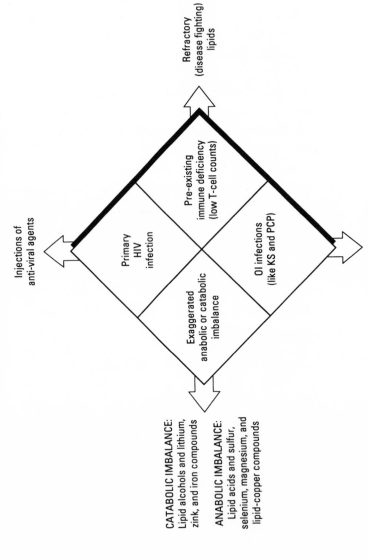

Revici's 4-Faceted Approach to Treating HIV

Injections of
anti-viral agents

Refractory
(disease fighting)
lipids

Pre-existing
immune deficiency
(low T-cell counts)

Primary
HIV
infection

OI infections
(like KS and PCP)

Exaggerated
anabolic or catabolic
imbalance

Antibiotics, antimicrobial,
or antifungal agents

CATABOLIC IMBALANCE:
Lipid alcohols and lithium,
zink, and iron compounds

ANABOLIC IMBALANCE:
Lipid acids and sulfur,
selenium, magnesium, and
lipid-copper compounds

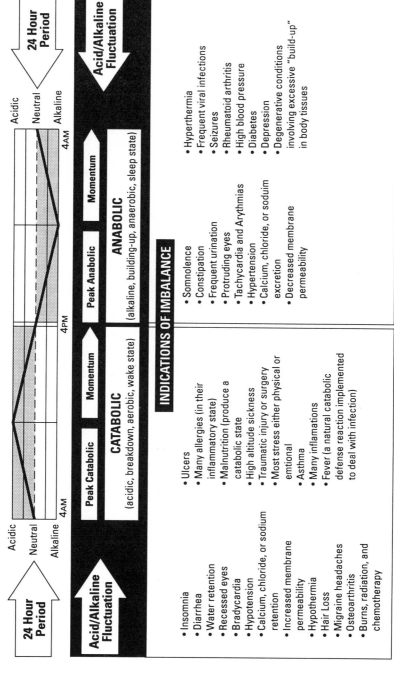

The Balance of Anabolic and Catabolic Forces Within the Body

Revici's Biological Aspect of the Periodic Table

CATIONIC — **ANIONIC** — **INERT**

Periods	Organizational Levels (ORBITAL)	I-A ANA.	II-A CATA.	III-B CATA.	IV-B ANA.	V-B CATA.	VI-B ANA.	VII-B CATA.	VIII-B ANA.	VIII-B CATA.	VIII-B ANA.	I-B CATA.	II-B ANA.	III-A ANA.	IV-A CATA.	V-A ANA.	VI-A CATA.	VII-A ANA.	INERT
1		1 H																1 H	2 He
2	Systemic	3 Li	4 Be											5 B	6 C	7 N	8 O	9 F	10 Ne
3	Metazoic	11 Na	12 Mg											13 Al	14 Si	15 P	16 S	17 Cl	18 Ar
4	Cellular (2)	19 K	20 Ca	21 Sc	22 Ti	23 V	24 Cr	25 Mn	26 Fe	27 Co	28 Ni	29 Cu	30 Zn	31 Ga	32 Ge	33 As	34 Se	35 Br	36 Kr
5	Nuclear (2-8)	37 Rb	38 Sr	39 Y	40 Zr	41 Nb	42 Mo	43 Tc	44 Ru	45 Rh	46 Pd	47 Ag	48 Cd	49 In	50 Sn	51 Sb	52 Te	53 I	54 Xe
6	Subnuclear (2-8-18)	55 Cs	56 Ba	57 La	72 Hf	73 Ta	74 W	75 Re	76 Os	77 Ir	78 Pt	79 Au	80 Hg	81 Tl	82 Pb	83 Bi	84 Po	85 A	86 Rn
7	Primary (2-8-18-32)	87 Fr	88 Ra	89 Ac															

Transition Metals

Rare Earth Metals

Lanthanides:

58 Ce ANA.	59 Pr CATA.	60 Nd ANA.	61 Pm CATA.	62 Sm ANA.	63 Eu CATA.	64 Gd ANA.	65 Tb CATA.	66 Dy ANA.	67 Ho CATA.	68 Er ANA.	69 Tm CATA.	70 Yb CATA.	71 Lu ANA.

Actinides:

90 Th	91 Pa	92 U	93 Np	94 Pu	95 Am	96 Cm	97 Bk	98 Cf	99 Es	100 Fm	101 Md	102 No	103 Lr

KEY

CATA. Anabolic or Catabolic
79 Atomic Number
Au Atomic Symbol

354

ABOUT THE AUTHOR

William Kelley Eidem is a free-lance writer. He has traveled thousands of miles, interviewed hundreds of people and read thousands of pages of documents to prepare this book. He is a graduate of the University of Maryland and lives in the Washington, D.C. area.

THE REVICI HONOR

To commemorate outstanding achievement in the field of medicine, the author is establishing a fund in the name of Emanuel Revici, M.D. Ten percent of the author's royalties will go to support this fund. If you wish to contribute to this prize award, please make your check payable to "The Revici Honor" and send to:

> The Revici Honor
> c/o William Kelley Eidem
> 4938 Hampden Lane #185
> Bethesda, MD 20815